KETO FOR WOMEN

This Book Includes : "Keto Diet Cookbook + Keto Diet For Women

Sara Clark

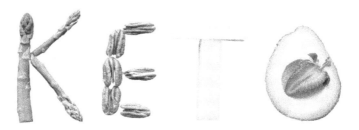

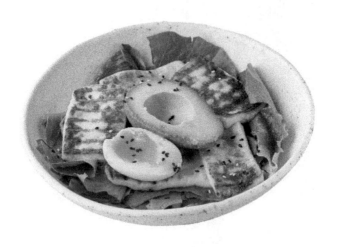

information is without a contract or any type of guarantee assurance.

The trademarks used are without any consent, and the publication of the trademark is without permission or backing by the trademark owner. All trademarks and brands within this book are for clarifying purposes only and are owned by the owners themselves, not affiliated with this document.

KETO DIET COOKBOOK

Contents

KETO DIET FOR WOMEN

Contents

KETO DIET COOKBOOK

An Effective Guide for Women with Delicious and Easy Recipes for Wieght Loss

By Jason Smith

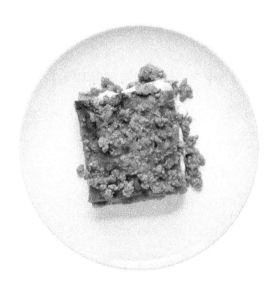

In no way is it legal to reproduce, duplicate, or transmit any part of this document in either electronic means or in printed format. Recording of this publication is strictly prohibited and any storage of this document is not allowed unless with written permission from the publisher. All rights reserved.

The information provided herein is stated to be truthful and consistent, in that any liability, in terms of inattention or otherwise, by any usage or abuse of any policies, processes, or directions contained within is the solitary and utter responsibility of the recipient reader. Under no circumstances will any legal responsibility or blame be held against the publisher for any reparation, damages, or monetary loss due to the information herein, either directly or indirectly.

Respective authors own all copyrights not held by the publisher.

The information herein is offered for informational purposes solely, and is universal as so. The presentation of the information is without contract or any type of guarantee assurance. The trademarks that are used are without any consent, and the publication of the trademark is without permission or backing by the trademark owner. All trademarks and brands within this book are for clarifying purposes only and are the owned by the owners themselves, not affiliated with this document.

Introduction

The Keto diet is a diet that is low in carbohydrates. In this diet, a person takes most of the calories from proteins and fats than from carbs. High carb, processed and sugary foods like candies, desserts, white bread and pasta are removed from the diet. If you take fewer grams of carbs in a day, your body systems don't have enough sugar to make energy. And in the keto diet, starts making energy by using ketones. To enter into the phase of ketosis, your body needs three to four days. Your fat starts melting then, and this helps you in losing weight. This diet emphasizes fat reduction rather than health benefits is a keto diet. People utilize a keto diet mostly to reduce weight, although it may help treat some problems like cardiac issues, neurological issues, epilepsy, PCOS etc. Insulin is a body hormone that helps glucose to be utilized or processed within the body as food. Keto diets allow you easily burn this food, so you do not have to store it. These lower insulin levels will help shield you against some forms of cancer or even delay cancerous cell development. It seems odd that a diet that is high in fats increases good cholesterol levels and lowers bad cholesterol levels. But the keto diet does it. It may be that the reduced insulin levels arising from the keto diet may inhibit the body from generating more cholesterol. It ensures that you are less likely to experience elevated blood pressure, cardiac disease, damaged arteries, and other medical problems. It has shown good results for acne-prone skin. This skin condition has been related to increased carbohydrate consumption, so cutting down on them helps. Reduction in insulin that a keto diet can cause also helps in avoiding breakouts. Diets low in carbs tend to keep blood pressure levels lower and in this way, it is good for hypertensive patients. It also helps diabetic patients in keep sugar levels low and insulin regulation. Keto diets have improved the regulation of seizures induced by this disease. Hence it is good for patients with epilepsy. It has also shown good results in patients with neurological conditions like Parkinson's, Alzheimer's etc. It is also helpful for sleep apnea and insomnia. Ketones your body produces in ketosis help shield your brain cells from injury. It also helps women with PCOS and fertility issues. It improves hormone levels and endocrine health. Other lifestyle improvements, such as working out, losing weight, and keto diets, help balance your hormone levels. It also helps athletes in building endurance, strength and cardiopulmonary fitness. Along with improving cardiovascular health, it also helps in building cardiopulmonary endurance and fitness. It has its advantages and disadvantages. There's a debate about its pros and cons everywhere. This book discusses how it impacts older women and health and why women should go for it.

Chapter 1: Basics of a Keto Diet

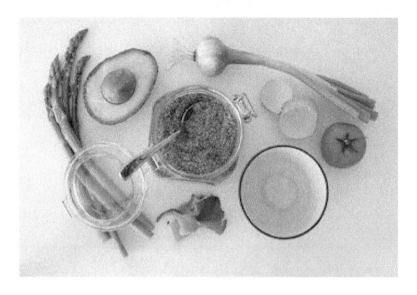

The keto diet is a low-carb and high-fat diet that has multiple health benefits. Studies suggest that a Keto diet can reduce the likelihood of contracting epilepsy, diabetes, cancer, Alzheimer's and other diseases. This chapter is a beginner's guide to the keto diet. In this type of diet, you cut on carbs as much as you can. It resembles other diets in many ways. It reduces carbohydrate consumption and substitutes it with fat. Ketosis is a metabolic condition of burning body fat for energy. When fat burning is effective, the body generates tonnes of energy. Ketogenic diets can induce substantial decreases in blood sugar and insulin levels. And as a result, a person loses weight. It reduces sugar and insulin levels, changing the body's metabolism to more fat and ketones.

1.1 Types of Keto Diets

There are many forms of the ketogenic diet. It is a rather low carb, high fat and mild protein diet. The cyclical keto diet includes five days fast accompanied by a two-day feast. A targeted ketogenic diet helps you to incorporate carbohydrates around workouts.Only the normal and high protein ketogenic diets have been studied. Ketogenic diets are more complex approaches used mainly by bodybuilders and athletes.

Standard Keto Diet

In this diet, you take only 5 to 10 percent carbs, 15 to 20 percent proteins and 75 percent fats. You schedule all meals and snacks around fat, such as ghee, olives, avocados, meat, sugar and fish on the regular keto diet. To change your metabolism such that it burns fat as food, you should consume more grams of fat a day than what you were taking before. You ought to cut the carbohydrates. Eat more greens and vegetables that are not rich in starch. Have fruits that have fewer carbs, such as melons or berries. Consume a moderate amount of proteins. You can get proteins by eating fish, eggs and meat etc.

Targeted Keto Diet

In this type of diet, you consume 20 percent proteins and 70 percent fat. This diet is common among athletes and healthy individuals who live a healthy lifestyle. It is important to consume 25 to 35 grams of carbohydrates directly before and after exercises to better heal from exercise. Many of the better choices are grains, fruits or other nutrition items. They are easily burnt off as fuel and do not end in fat accumulation or weight gain.

Cyclic Keto Diet

In this type of diet, there are days when you consume 20 percent proteins and 75 to 80 percent fats, followed by days where you consume 50 percent proteins and only 25 percent fats. This keto cycling is a way to cycle in and out of ketosis while enjoying a more healthy lifestyle on the days when you eat more proteins and fewer fats. We suggest you take fruits, dairy items, less starchy vegetables, and whole grains rather than processed or sugary foods on the off days.

High Protein Keto Diet

In this diet, you consume only 10 percent carbs, 30 percent proteins and 60 percent fats. Have proteins from beef, meat, fish and eggs. Keep carbs for only 5 to 10 percent of the total daily calorie intake. Many people find this type simpler to adopt. In this way, proteins convert into glucose for energy, but ketosis doesn't take place. However, such diets that are high in proteins help in weight loss.

1.2 What is ketosis?

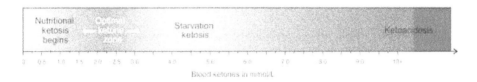

Ketosis is a metabolic condition in which the body utilizes fat for food. You decrease your carb intake, limiting the body's glucose availability, the primary source of sugar for the cells. Ketosis can be accomplished by adopting a ketogenic diet. Consume fewer carbs in a day; however, consume healthier fats like beef, eggs, seafood, nuts, and oils. Protein intake is therefore quite significant. Protein takes up a lot of space in the digestive tract, which limits ketone production. Intermittent fasting will help you get into ketosis quicker. There are several intermittent fasting ways, although the most popular is to eat for about eight hours a day and fast for the rest of the day. Keto diets help you in losing weight. The possible side effects involve the dry mouth, more urination, elevated thirst and reduced appetite.

1.3 Benefits of Keto Diet

A ketogenic diet is an easy way to reduce weight and decrease the risk levels for illness. It can be almost as beneficial as a low-fat diet. It is not as challenging to manage because it does not require calorie tracking or weighing food. A study has shown low carb diets are more successful for long-term weight reduction than low-fat diets. People who follow keto diets have shown to have fewer blood pressure problems. In a report, older adults who adopted a ketogenic diet lost five times as much weight as those who followed a low-fat diet. Ketones reduce blood sugar and increased insulin sensitivity, which plays a key role in this.

- Diabetes is characterized by elevated blood pressure levels and reduced insulin regulation. The Keto diet helps in managing sugar levels and insulin regulation. It also helps to lose extra weight healthily. Keto diets may contribute to major health benefits for people with diabetes.

- Keto diets first came to be used for curing neurological disorders. However, now it has proven effects across a wide range of various health problems.

- It also helps in treating heart problems. Keto diet increases good cholesterol levels, decreases blood pressure and blood sugar levels.

- Children and adults on the ketogenic diet also show substantial declines in seizures.

- There is also tentative proof that the diet is an effective cure for cancer.

- The keto diet could benefit. Alzheimer's patients and delay its progression.

- A study showed that the keto diet could help improve symptoms of Parkinson's disease.

- The keto diet may help with insulin levels, which could play a key role in treating Polycystic Ovarian Syndrome.

- A keto diet can help to manage many metabolic, neurological, or insulin-related diseases.

1.4 What not to eat in a Keto Diet

Foods rich in carbs should be reduced. You can only have a small number of carbs in a day, which is only 5 to 20 percent of the daily calorie intake. Don't eat the following items:

- Processed foods

- Sugary items

- Vegetables rich in starch

- Noodles

- Strawberries

- Mayonnaise

- Sauces like ketchup or barbecue sauce

- Soft drinks

- Wine, Alcohol

- Candies, Sweeteners

- Desserts

- Pasta

- Rice

1.5 What to eat when on a Keto Diet

Eat more proteins and fewer carbs. Mostly you eat foods that have more fat in them. Here are some foods that you should consume to complete your daily calorie intake.

- Beef, Meat, Fish, Eggs.

- Butter or cream.

- All types of cheese.

- Nuts like walnuts and almonds.

- Seeds like chia, flaxseeds, pumpkin etc.

- Olive, Avocado, Coconut oil.

- Low carb, less starchy vegetables

A keto diet can be used to reduce weight, regulate blood pressure, and boost fitness. You can consume many healthy, delicious and flexible foods that fit into your everyday carb range. Include keto-friendly ingredients in your daily meals.

Seafood

Shellfish are keto-friendly ingredients. Fish is high in B vitamins,

potassium, and selenium yet practically carb-free. However, the carbohydrates in various forms of shellfish vary. Even though shellfish may be on a ketogenic diet, it is essential to account for the carbs when staying within a range. Fish rich in omega-3 fats have been shown to reduce insulin levels and improve insulin sensitivity in overweight and obese people. Fish consumption has been related to reduce the risk of illness and increased comprehension. It is advised to consume at least one seafood meal each week. Most forms of seafood have minimal to no carbs. Fish and shellfish have vitamins, nutrients, and omega-3s.

Avocados

Avocados are extremely nutritious. They are a decent source of potassium, an essential mineral that people do not get enough of. A higher potassium consumption will make the keto diet simpler. They help to improve and lower cholesterol and triglyceride levels.Avocados are rich in fiber and other nutrients, including potassium. They improve the cardiac and overall health of a person.

Low-carb Vegetables

Non-starchy vegetables have a limited number of calories and carbohydrates but contain multiple nutrients. When consumed, plant fiber is not digested or processed in the body. Because of this, you need to look at the digestible carbs count. Most veggies are poor in carbohydrates. One serving of starchy vegetables like beets, potatoes, yams etc., will bring you over your carb cap for the day. Plants include antioxidants that help defend against free radicals, which can trigger cell damage. Cruciferous crops, including cauliflower, kale and broccoli, can lower the risk of cancer and heart diseases. Consume avocado, broccoli, cabbage, asparagus, cauliflower, cucumber, lettuce, green beans, kale, eggplant, peppers, olives, spinach, tomatoes and zucchini etc.

Greek yogurt and cottage cheese

They are rich in protein and low in fat. Though they contain some carbs, you can still consume moderate quantities of them. Yogurt and cottage cheese have been found to suppress hunger and make them feel full. Some people like adding some sliced nuts to their smoothies to make them a bit richer. Both simple Greek yogurt and cottage cheese produce five grams of carbs. They can help reduce appetite and encourage fullness.

Cheese

There are several forms of cheese like feta, cheddar, mozzarella etc. They are rich in fat and low in carbs, making them suitable for a keto diet. Cheese includes saturated fat, but no research has shown that it increases the risk of heart failure. Some research indicates that cheese may help protect against heart disease. One ounce of cheddar cheese contains one gram of calories, proteins, and calcium. Cheese has been related to weight reduction. Also, frequently consuming cheese can help boost muscle mass and strength loss with aging. Cheese includes modest levels of protein, calcium, and healthy fatty acids.

Butter/cream

A balanced keto diet should contain butter and milk. One serving includes only some quantities of carbs. Cream and butter are thought to lead to cardiac failure owing to their high saturated fat content. Many major findings prove saturated fat is not related to cardiac problems. It is proposed that high-fat dairy consumption can help reduce cardiac failure and stroke risk. They are high in linoleic acid, the fatty acid that can encourage fat loss. They are low in calories, and they tend to have a neutral or positive impact on cardiac protection.

Poultry

Meats and eggs are essential ingredients of a keto diet. Fresh meat and poultry are high in B vitamins and other essential minerals. They are a decent source of high-quality protein that retains muscle mass during a very low carb diet. They help in improving cholesterol levels. The safest meat options are grass-fed livestock meat because it is rich in omega-3 fatty acids, conjugated acid, and antioxidants. Eggs are one of the healthiest items. They have more proteins and fewer carbs. Eggs may also activate hormones that enhance sensations of fullness and satiety. It also helps to protect eyesight. Egg yolks contain plenty of cholesterol, so they don't increase cholesterol levels among most people. Eggs reduce the amount of bad cholesterol in the body, which reduces the risk of heart diseases.

Coconuts

Coconut oil renders a huge part of a keto diet. It includes triglycerides taken up immediately by the liver and used as a rapid supply of nutrition. In reality, coconut oil may increase the ketone levels in the body. Coconut oil can help with weight loss and get rid of belly fat.

Oils

Olive oil offers remarkable health benefits. It is rich in omega-3 fatty acids that have been proven to lower heart attack risk factors. Virgin olive oil also includes antioxidants. This has shown a way to minimize inflammation and enhance artery function and hence improves cardiac health. It has no carbs as a fat source. It is an excellent basis for dressings and mayonnaise. Extra-virgin olive oil is rich in monounsaturated fats and antioxidants. It's perfect for salad dressings and cooking.

Nuts/Seeds

Nuts and seeds are balanced snacks. Eating nuts may help avoid cardiac failure, cancers, tumors, obesity, and many other chronic diseases. Nuts and seeds are rich in fiber and absorb fewer calories overall. You can have the following nuts or seeds:

- Almonds

- Walnuts

- Chia seeds

- Pumpkin seeds

- Flaxseeds

Nuts and seeds are heart-healthy, rich in fiber, and can contribute to healthier aging.

Berries

Fruits cannot be consumed on a keto diet, although berries are permitted. Berries are poor in carbohydrates and fiber. In reality, raspberries and blackberries produce a lot of fiber. These tiny fruits are full of antioxidants that combat inflammation and defend against diseases.

Coffee/Tea

Coffee and tea are carb-free beverages. The caffeine in these beverages might boost physical performance and mood. Coffee and tea drinkers have been found to have a decreased chance of diabetes. The higher the caffeine consumption, the lower the chance of developing diabetes. Coffee and tea will help improve your metabolic rate, as well as physical and mental efficiency.

Dark chocolate and Cocoa powder

Dark chocolate and cocoa produce antioxidant amounts. In reality, cocoa contains at least as much antioxidant activity as blueberries. Dark chocolate has flavanols, which can aid reduce blood pressure and maintain veins and arteries safe. Consuming chocolate should be part of a ketogenic diet. It is necessary to select dark chocolate that contains at least seventy percent cocoa. Dark chocolate and cocoa can lower the risk of heart disease.

1.6 Sample Diet Meal Plan

In the keto diet, you take fewer carbs, moderate proteins and high fats. Here is a sample keto diet meal plan for one week.

Day One:

- Have egg muffins and fruits for Breakfast.

- Have vegetable or chicken salad with some cheese for Lunch.

- Have a grilled fish with butter for Dinner.

Day Two:

- Have an omelet with veggies for Breakfast.

- Have a banana and peanut butter smoothie with almond milk for Lunch. You can use chocolate powder or stevia sugar for taste.

- Have cheese and salsa tacos for Dinner.

Day Three:

- Have chia pudding with berries and coconut for Breakfast.

- Have an avocado sandwich for Lunch.

- Have pork with broccoli and salad for Dinner.

Day Four:

- Have an omelet made up of chilies, tomato, onion, salsa and other spices for Breakfast.

- Have some almonds or other nuts for Lunch.

- Have chicken filled with cream and cheese with some vegetables like broccoli or zucchini for Dinner.

Day Five:

- Have greek yogurt with berries, chocolate and cocoa powder for Breakfast.
- Make beef or chicken lettuce wrap for Lunch.
- Have some mixed vegetables for Dinner.

Day Six:

- Have pancakes with berries and other fruits for Breakfast.
- Have any salad or zucchini noodles for Lunch.
- Have fried fish with veggies or nuts for Dinner.

Day Seven:

- Have an egg with mushrooms for Breakfast.
- Have low carb chicken with vegetables for Lunch.
- Have spaghetti with vegetables for Dinner.

Try to change vegetables and meat with various forms that have different foods and health benefits. In this way, you won't ever get bored of eating such food. Plan your meals and make them easy and fun for yourself. Explore your options and try new recipes. You will consume several balanced foods on a ketogenic diet. Perfect keto snacks contain bits of beef, fish, eggs, cheese, fruits, olives, walnuts, almonds, vegetables, olives and dark chocolate.

1.7 Tips for Keto Diet

It is simpler to initiate the ketogenic diet, but it is hard to stay consistent with it. You need to know about the tricks that will help you in staying motivated and consistent. Here are few tips for that:

- Always look at the calorie count of what food you are consuming. Check how many proteins, fats or carbs it has in it.

- Plan your meals. It will also save you some time.

- Try new recipes and make your keto meals more interesting.

- Search recipes on blogs or videos etc. Find low-carb and high-fat recipes.

- Whenever you go out, take your keto snacks with you. It will help you satisfy your cravings.

- Reading food labeling, preparing your meals accordingly, and carrying your snacks will make keeping to the keto diet even simpler.

- If you go to any restaurant, have beef or fish, or have egg-based dishes.

- Choose an egg-based recipe for your main course. Get greens instead of starches, and eat a slice of cheese.

1.8 Side effects of Keto Diet

A keto diet is generally suitable for most healthy people but can have certain side effects. Some of them are written below:

- Diarrhea, nausea, constipation, and vomiting.

- Fatigue, lack of concentration.

- Increase in appetite or cravings.

- Insomnia or other sleep problems.

You should reduce back on the sugar consumption to minimize sugar cravings. It can help you lose more fat until you remove carbs. A ketogenic diet can also induce improvements in the water and mineral content of the body. It's important to keep eating before you're complete and not limiting calories too much. It functions well without calorie limitation. Adverse effects of the ketogenic diet may reduce with time. Start slowly and move

towards a healthy diet.

However, in the long run, the keto diet can

have certain harmful consequences, including chances of the following:

- Low blood protein.
- Fat deposits in stomach.
- Kidney stones.
- Mineral deposition.

If you have serious medical problems, then contact your doctor before starting a keto diet. A keto diet can benefit people with:.

- Obesity
- Diabetes
- Cardiac problems
- Athletes

The extremely low carb, high-fat diet has proven promise for weight reduction, diabetes, and epilepsy. There is also proof that it can aid with certain tumors, Alzheimer's disease, and other diseases. Despite these issues, more study is required on the diet's long-term protection and effectiveness.

Chapter 2: Why you should choose Keto Diet?

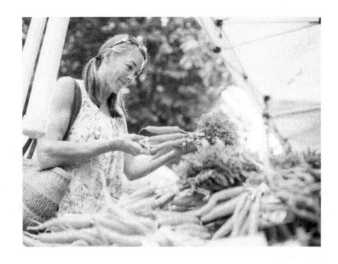

A keto diet is an eating pattern based on foods with plenty of good fats, sufficient nutrition, and relatively few carbs. The aim is to get more calories from fat than from carbs. By depleting the body of its sugar supplies, this diet functions. As a consequence, fat for energy can continue to break down. This results in the production of ketones named molecules that the body uses for food. It may also contribute to losing weight as the body burns fat.

2.1 How does this diet work?

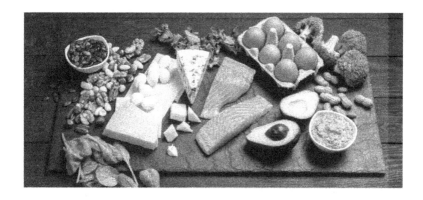

The keto diet aims to push your body to burn ketones for food instead of depending on sugar from carbohydrates (such as legumes, vegetables, grains and fruits). As you know, the human body is primarily fuelled by glucose, which we obtain by carbohydrates such as rice, cereal, pasta, bread etc. Our digestive system converts nutrients into sugar, named glucose, which is the element that our bodies use to produce energy. But when the body is not getting enough carb-rich foods, it makes energy by a different mechanism, and one such mechanism is called ketosis. The body then generates energy from fat. The liver converts fats into ketone products. If you deprive the body of food, either by eating or adopting a very low carb diet, the body joins the physiological process. To enter ketosis, the carb consumption needs to be reduced to fewer than 5 to 10 percent in a day, which is the key guideline in the low-carb diet. Even while you're attempting to adopt the low-carb diet, think of this as an estimate. You will have about five to ten percent of your daily calories from carbs in a keto diet. Your diet will consist of about fifteen percent of your daily calories from protein and about seventy-five percent of your daily calories coming from fat. You will be receiving much of your daily calories from eggs, meat, vegetables and cheese.

Burning fat by ketosis is perfect for losing weight. It normally takes a few days to attain ketosis. Excess protein intake may interact with ketosis. You are advised to consume the fat you want, regardless of the source, such as cheese, butter, meat, eggs, olive oil, until you feel satisfied when practicing keto. Fatty foods may increase nausea for some and diarrhea for others. In addition to possible physical pain, it might not be mentally convenient for everyone. Keto diet is also a limited diet that usually isn't a safe option for those with eating or other disorders. Just like any restrictive diet, a keto diet can be difficult to stay consistent with. To continue in ketosis, it might be important to reduce cultural food consumption in the diet. Preventing carbs every day involves cooking and planning meals before time.

2.2 Weight loss with Keto Diet

An effective, long-lasting weight loss is often the outcome of several variables such as:

- A balanced diet
- Physical exercise
- Sleep
- Stress management
- Other medical conditions

In the first few weeks, some people lose some pounds. They need to get that is just the water weight. The keto diet can be a diuretic that causes water loss from muscles, fat, and liver cells due to glycogen's storing.

Although weight loss may be your primary target, it is vital to consider the two factors; turning your short-term diet into a long-term lifestyle and testing important health biomarkers. The weight you lose will only be for a short period if they are overlooked.

Hold a thirty percent or lower calorie deficit. When you consume fewer calories than the body requires to maintain its weight, you'll lose weight. If your calorie deficiency is over thirty percent, though, you are more prone to get hungry and slow down your metabolism and recover your weight if you do not feed. Eat enough protein. Even if you don't lift the weight, your keto diet needs to consume a decent protein amount. When you satisfy your protein requirements, you'll lower your appetite, eat more calories and help maintain muscle fat, helping to shed weight while you look and feel better.

And even though ketogenic diets seem good for healthier people in the short term, there is still a lack of long-term dietary evidence. Complications of a keto diet are nausea, diarrhea, constipation, gastrointestinal problems, stomach or kidney stones, pancreas issues and calcium deficiency.

2.3 Keto Diet for Athletes

Athletes also encourage the keto diet to improve fat metabolism. It is often said that carbs limit how fast or far you can go as an athlete. In other words, when it comes to athletic success lasting up to three hours, your body's capacity to use fat for energy supply isn't important. In certain studies, ketogenic diets' success has been detrimental, possibly due to the additional oxygen necessary if your body has to depend on fat for energy. Some claim that since athletes will consume what they want, the fat consumption may not have an adverse effect. Some research has shown negative health effects of diets high in dietary fat, particularly saturated fat, including a rise in heart disease and diabetes risk.

2.4 Keto diet for Skin Problems

Acne has many common reasons and can link with what food you are eating and blood sugar levels in certain persons. Consuming a diet rich in processed and refined carbohydrates can change the equilibrium of intestinal bacteria and cause major changes in blood sugar levels, both of which can adversely affect the skin's health.

According to some reports, a keto diet may alleviate acne symptoms in certain individuals by reducing carb intake.

2.5 Keto diet for Health Problems

Cancer

It can decrease the risk of a certain type of cancer. The implications of the keto diet have been studied by experts to potentially avoid or even cure such cancers. One research showed that in patients with some diseases, a keto diet could be a healthy and complementary way to be used in addition to radiation and chemotherapy. This is because it can cause more oxidative stress in cancer cells than in regular cells, allowing them to die.It has also been indicated that it may also reduce the possibility of diabetic complications since the keto diet decreases blood sugar levels. Insulin is a blood sugar balance hormone that can be linked to certain cancers. Researchers need to perform further trials to truly appreciate the keto diet's possible effects on cancer prevention and treatment.

Cardiac Issues

A Keto diet may enhance cardiac health. When an individual practices a keto diet, selecting nutritious foods is important. Studies have shown that consuming healthier fats, such as avocados, may boost heart protection by reducing cholesterol deposition in arteries or veins. Keto diet improves the storage and regulation of good cholesterol and prevents the storage of bad cholesterol. Raised cholesterol levels affect human health and generally cause heart problems. Being on a keto diet reduces the risk of the occurrence of heart problems. However, the beneficial benefits of the diet on cardiac health rely on its consistency. Thus, when adopting the keto diet, it is essential to consume nutritionally balanced food.

Brain Problems

Studies have shown that ketones produced by ketosis have positive effects on brain health and neurons. They help in protecting neurons. Nerve cells work in a better way. That's why the keto diet has shown positive results in patients with Alzheimer's or Parkinson's disease for this cause. However, more research needs to be done in this area. In a keto diet, the fat, protein, and carbs ratio changes how the body absorbs nutrition, culminating in ketosis. Ketosis is a biochemical mechanism during which ketone the body uses bodies for food. Ketosis in people with epilepsy, particularly those who have not adapted to other types of care, may minimize seizures. More study is required into how effective this is, as it seems to have the biggest influence on children who have seizures. The keto diet is shown to minimize epilepsy symptoms.

Keto Diet for Polycystic Ovarian Syndrome

A hormonal disease that may contribute to cysts' formation in ovaries, excess production of male hormones and ovulatory failure is polycystic ovary syndrome. A high-carb diet can trigger adverse effects in such women, such as skin problems and weight gain. It has been reported that women with this condition had shown good results when they followed the keto diet.

- It has helped in losing weight.

- It has regulated hormone levels.

- It improves blood sugar and insulin levels.

2.6 General Guidelines for Keto diet

It is necessary to negotiate with a doctor, dietitian, or trustworthy healthcare professional for every planned diet plan, especially for individuals attempting to handle a health condition or disease. To guarantee that the keto diet is a healthy eating pattern, individuals trying to start the keto diet can contact a doctor to verify whether they have diabetes, hypoglycemia, cardiac illness, or other health

46

problems. Bear in mind that reports are incomplete on the long-term benefits of the keto diet. It is uncertain if it is more effective than less healthy eating habits to sustain this lifestyle for longer periods. A ketogenic diet restricts carbs or seriously reduces them. Individuals can follow a diet that contains several nutrient-dense, fibrous carbohydrates, such as fruits and less starchy vegetables, together with balanced protein sources and healthier fats, for a less restrictive dietary method.

Lifestyle changes with Keto Diet

Keto diet often requires lifestyle changes, as with any diet program. The goods that have added sugar are strongly prohibited because they provide nothing in the way of nutrients. You cannot have sugary or processed items in this diet as soft drinks, cakes, biscuits, desserts, white bread, sugar snacks, burgers, popcorns etc., because they are high in carbs, they make ketosis slow. The Keto diet regulates insulin and sugar levels. A reduction in insulin will impair sodium accumulation, which allows it easier for sodium and fluids to excrete. It also helps in lowering blood pressure. Like all the other diets, the ketogenic diet is not a special solution to both our wishes and desires of wellbeing and weight. It may be pleasant for some people, especially in the first few weeks, but it will not be easy for everyone.

But it is a good way to lose weight for a long period. Adherence and satisfaction are the two important dietary improvement methods that can yield any meal's greatest results. Make your meals fun and tasty. It is advised to treat cardiac issues by raising your fiber amount and restricting your saturated fat consumption. Although research on saturated fat is evolving, it is ideal for fiber sources and unsaturated fats that reduce the risk of heart disease and allow a more healthy intake of nutrients.

You need to take these factors into account to build a lifestyle that helps you sustain your weight loss success and optimize your health:

- Meal options

- Lifestyle changes

- Social interactions

- Purpose of the following diet

We are emotionally motivated people, and food is one of the most strong generators of emotion. Such dietary choices continuously inspire you in your food setting, from your kitchen to your office and all in between. Sadly, much of our food environments influence us to make far tougher choices than decisions that help us remain safe. It is not just desired that it is key to stop these bad food choices. Instead of that, we need to make good choices.

In other terms, both the subconscious and the aware facets of your mind will affect you in making good decisions and maintaining your lifetime loss.

- Remove all the processed and sugary food items from your home.

- Eat-in portions and less amount.

- Take nutritious snacks with you.

- Make your meals at home.

- When eating out, go for healthier choices.

- Track your calorie count for everyday meals.

While a diet can be held and outcomes collected for a few months, your lifestyle is predominant on a long-term basis. Therefore you must discuss your entire lifestyle before entering a new diet and how it impacts your life. Start where you really are and adjust slowly. For starters, don't attempt running a marathon or suddenly lift hundreds of pounds. Increase your health in a manageable and friendly manner. It isn't easy to make significant dietary changes, especially when you do it alone. There will be days when you'll fail to find motivation, hours of questioning why you cannot lose weight more easily. You have to start making changes to your current lifestyle to render your short-term weight reduction a long-term result. Transform the present lifestyle into a healthy one by making little progressive improvements that can quickly be turned into new behaviors.

Chapter 3: Keto Diet for Women over Fifty years of Age

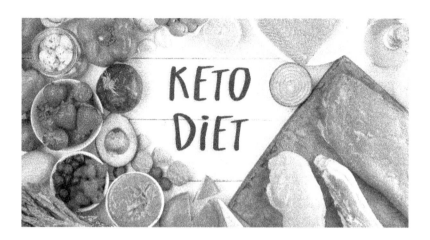

If you're a female above fifty years of age, you may be much keener in losing weight as compared to your thirties. In old age, your metabolism becomes slow, and it increases your weight. Slower metabolism and a passive lifestyle causes muscle damage and will render weight gain incredibly challenging. There are various dietary options for losing those extra pounds, but the ketogenic diet was recently one of the most common and famous ones.

3.1 Why should women go for Keto Diet?

A Ketogenic diet is intended to minimize calories and raise the amount of fat you consume to make the body more effective in burning its fat and losing weight. Keto diets improve the overall well-being of a person. Keto foods have enabled many women to get rid of extra fat or weight without starving themselves. It has shown positive effects in women with diabetes, heart and hormonal problems. When your blood sugar level decreases because of ketosis, your body releases ketone molecules and uses them to generate energy for the body. Keto molecules are created when carbohydrate consumption is decreased and protein consumption is in a moderate quantity. When your body starts using ketones for energy production, it means it has entered ketosis. In certain situations, this causes the body to significantly burn fat, which helps lose weight. This not helps you to lose weight, but it also reduces cravings.

3.2 Is it safe for women over fifty years?

It depends on a variety of variables that a Ketogenic diet is good for women above fifty years of age or not. This diet may have a variety of advantages, particularly for losing weight. If you don't have serious medical problems, then it is safe to go for this diet type. Eat everything in a balanced way and keep check of its nutritional figures. Don't exceed the daily calorie count. The best way to eat healthy food in a balanced way is literally by adhering to whole grains, largely because this is a suitable strategy. You will find it hard to stick to this diet initially, but you'll get used to it with time.

How Keto diet has positive results?

In this diet, you limit carb intake to the stage when your body starts ketosis and burns fat rather than sugar for energy production. A slow metabolism can be treated by having a balanced diet. After thirty years of age, most of the women lose muscle mass. As they grow older, their bones and muscles become weaker every day. When you take enough proteins in this diet, it helps you in improving muscle function. Consuming fat from good foods helps control your food cravings, so you don't feel an urge to cheat on the keto diet. You can stick to this diet type for a long period and improve your health gradually. It balances your sugar and cholesterol levels. It has also been shown to treat arthritic pain in women, treats acne, and improves hair condition.

3.3 Guidelines for women following Keto Diet

Certain research suggests that a few causing factors for cardiac issues, involving storage of bad cholesterol, can be elevated by using the keto diet. Studies suggest that the keto diet improves cardiac protective good cholesterol levels and lowers bad cholesterol levels, although others have shown that the keto diet substantially boosts cholesterol levels. While it has been seen that the keto diet can improve some causative factors for cardiac failure, further study is required to establish if this type of diet can improve or lessen the occurrence of cardiac problems and further study its overall effects on human health.

Who shouldn't go for the Keto diet?

The keto diet is not suitable for some women because of its stringent and hard-to-retain food nutrient ratio. Here is a list of women who shouldn't go for the keto diet:

- Alcoholic women.

- Women who have type 1 diabetes.

- Women with creatinine or vitamin deficiency.

- Women with blood disorders.

- Women with eating disorders.

- Pregnant or women who are breastfeeding their newborns.

- Women with kidney stones, pancreas or liver problems.

There are several variables to remember when trying the keto diet, in addition to the conditions mentioned here. The keto diet can trigger painful signs that are recognized as ketogenic flu. It causes diarrhea, nausea, constipation or fatigue etc. These signs usually recover after some days or a week.

Who should go for the Keto Diet?

It is required to weigh the good and bad implications of a keto diet. Also, keep your medical condition in mind before starting any diet plan. Results of diet depend on these factors. For instance, for an asthmatic, obese woman and is facing difficulty maintaining her sugar levels by using dietary changes, the keto diet might be a good option. The keto diet can also be beneficial for females who are obese or who have hormonal issues. Research has shown that the ketogenic diet can improve the health of women with polycystic ovaries. It helps them in losing weight, managing hormones and improves reproductive health as a result. It's often recommended to follow a dietary plan abundant in healthy food options that can be preserved based on your fitness and nutritional requirements. As the ketogenic diet is an extremely low-carb diet, and its success relies on preserving ketones, it is advised to practice this plan only while consulting with a trained health provider. If you are involved in carrying out a keto diet, talk to a care practitioner or a licensed nutritionist.

3.4 Advantages of Ketogenic Diet for Females

- It gives you a positive mindset and clarity. When you are on a keto diet, your brain function improves, and keto molecules clean your brain cells. It improves your brain's cognitive performance. It also helps in fighting depression and anxiety issues.

- It reduces mood swings. It gives your mind a healthy and positive approach and you generally feel happy. Sugar level imbalances mostly cause mood swings and anger issues. It controls sugar and insulin levels and hence helps in keeping your overall health under control.

- By eating healthy and working out, you generally feel good. It boosts your self-esteem and helps you in living a better life. It improves energy levels, and you feel active throughout the day. The energy produced from keto molecules gives you more reliable energy than the one from sugar molecules.

- It helps in reducing sugar and food cravings by regulating your hormones. With imbalanced insulin levels, you feel hungry unnecessarily. When your sugar levels are balanced, your appetite is controlled, and your fat is burning because of ketosis. Fats make you feel full for a long period, and hence you don't binge on sugary foods.

- It helps you lose weight gradually and sustainably. You are eating healthy and nutritious food, which helps in curing many health problems and losing weight.

Workouts with Keto Diet

- Workout or walk for at least thirty minutes a day.

- Do strengthening exercises at least three days a week. They help in making your metabolism fast and help in losing weight.

- Set easy goals and progress gradually. Don't overtire your body. Start with doing exercise for two or three days a week for twenty to thirty minutes and then gradually increase the time and repetitions.

- Lifting weights also help in burning fat and losing fat.

3.5 Eating rules of a Keto Diet

Discover your options and keep track of what you are eating. You have to meet the daily calorie intake. Make sure you are taking fewer carbs, adequate proteins and more fats. It is important to enter the ketosis phase and sustain it for burning fat and losing weight. Balance your food plate and eat in portions. Your plate should have carbs, fats and proteins in a fixed amount. It's not that you completely get rid of carbs. The aim is to remove poor quality carbs such as starchy foods, packaged items and processed carbohydrates, which induce swelling, digestive problems, chemical imbalances and improve the quality of healthier fats in your body to teach your body to get rid of excess fat and harmful materials by the things you are having and energy storage.

It is a fairly major adjustment, and it can take time for the body to get used to this, so it's not surprising to feel some tiredness, mood swings and food cravings.

3.6 Supplements for Keto Diet

It's not mandatory to take Ketogenic pills to adopt this diet because you will completely get fantastic outcomes without using them, but they can assist you in losing weight and achieving your fitness goals quickly and effectively. Keto supplements help you in getting essential vitamins and minerals that you aren't getting from food. They reduce the keto diet risks, such as nausea, diarrhea, headaches and fatigue etc. Some of the supplements are described here:

- **Electrolytes:** The most effective approach to avoid ketogenic flu, such as signs of vomiting, exhaustion and fatigue, is to use a substitute. Your body can not absorb as much water while adapting to diet so that you can face the problem of dehydration. And even you are sweating out while working out but not taking enough water, then that's a problem. Make sure you are drinking more than enough water in a day. Drink a lot of water with electrolyte supplements in the morning. Take salty foods and the ones which are rich in iron, potassium and magnesium. Take zinc, magnesium and potassium supplements, which are substitutes for electrolytes and perform well with a ketogenic diet.

- **Probiotics:** They are essential for the digestive, immune, endocrine system and optimal health. They have good bacterial organisms that clean the gut area and improve gut functioning. They also make antibodies naturally and improve the functioning of neuron cells. It regulates hormone levels. It is a good vitamin and energy source for people following a keto diet.

- **Omega-3 supplements:** It is best to take them via supplements. They are needed for enhancing brain function. They are also seen to treat depression and anxiety issues. They decrease cholesterol deposition and improve heart health. They improve body mass index and help in losing weight. They reduce body inflammation mechanism by regulating sugar and cholesterol levels.

- **Magnesium supplements:** It helps in maintaining sugar and insulin levels of your body and improves immune function. It enhances the overall performance of the body's systems. Broccoli, pumpkin seeds and avocados are found to have adequate magnesium concentrations. So consume such foods to meet this need.

- **Collagen:** It is an integral component of the bodily tissues such as muscles, bones, skin, tendons and ligaments. Our body doesn't make it naturally, so it is important to take its supplements. It improves skin elasticity and makes you look young. It strengthens bones and keeps them in good shape. It protects your organs and joint structure.

- **Medium Chain Triglyceride Oils:** They are a good energy source when you are on a ketogenic diet. These triglycerides taken from food are converted into ketone molecules and are used to generate energy and burn fat. If you want to speed up fat burning and weight loss, you should use these supplements. They are tasteless; you can mix them in your coffee or take them with water.

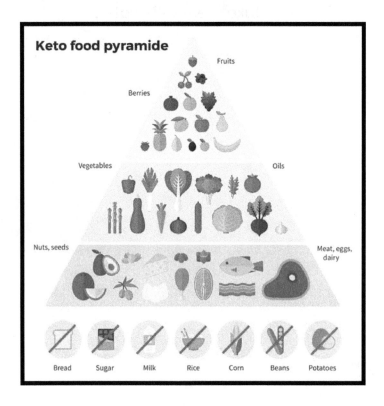

Keto diets are hard to stay consistent with because you are not only taking fewer calories than before, but you are also consuming fewer carbs. You won't get any results if you do not stay consistent with this diet. Your body needs to go into the ketosis phase to burn fat. However, this diet is a safer option because you aren't starving yourself. You are taking healthy and nutritious foods in a fixed pattern and quantity.

Here are some tips to speed up the process of fat burning and losing weight with the keto diet:

Consume extra fats for the first few weeks.

- It controls the working of your body systems to burn fat. It speeds up the working mechanism of mitochondria for the latest energy supply.

- It controls calorie intake and doesn't cause a calorie imbalance in the body.

- It offers therapeutic support for you. It's a smart way to remember that you can consume more fat and lose those extra pounds and that too in a healthy way.

- The body uses its own stored fats in fatty tissues and hence the volume of stored fat decreases and ketones burn them.

- The ones who want to gain weight should continue taking extra fats throughout their diet.

Take enough calories in a day.

- Don't try to overdo this diet. You are supposed to take the required amount of calories through carbs, fats and proteins.

- Eat-in small portions and take frequent meals. Just balance your calorie intake.

- Don't undereat or overeat. Eat until your hunger is satisfied.

Choose fasting or Keto diet.

- When mixing exceptionally low carb diets with prolonged fasting or continuously shortened feeding windows, people face many problems. They are either taking too low calories or too many calories.

- The purpose of the keto diet is to speed up fat burning by consuming a healthy diet. Somehow fasting does the same. But if you do both of these together, it causes many medical problems. It becomes hard to get the desired results.

- Introduce one change to your body at a time to allow your body a better understanding of the condition.

Take nutrient-rich foods.

- Have meat, beef, fish etc.

- Use olive oil or coconut oil.

- Use all types of cheese.

- Have salads or smoothies.

- Discover your food options and experiment with them.

- Have less starchy vegetables like broccoli, olives, avocadoes etc.

- Take proteins in moderate quantity from legumes and eggs etc.

Don't be too hard on yourself.

- In the start, you would have to push yourself to stick to this diet, but soon you will get used to it.

- For three to four weeks, staying consistent with keto is important as it works great for burning fat.

- Appreciate yourself through the process.

- It is important to keep your mindset positive for staying motivated.

- The Keto diet is important for strengthening your metabolism.

Monitor your body responses

- Taking fewer calories isn't always the solution. Often the body wants more time to feed, maybe more proteins or carbohydrates or protein in particular.

- It will take time for your body to understand and adapt itself to new mechanisms and energy pathways. It takes time to adjust to ketosis.

- Women are more vulnerable to metabolic or nutritional abnormalities, so they need to be careful about this diet.

- It is obvious that if you deprive your body of essential nutrients, then your body will suffer.

- Some diets, such as the ones for epilepsy, needs fewer proteins, so their diets have less number of proteins.

4.2 Common Keto Diet Mistakes and their Solutions

It may be challenging to understand what effects weight reduction. Keto diets are highly restrictive and a bit hard to stick to. You would have to mix different vegetables on this diet, restrict starchy vegetables, and don't use nuts, drinks, sugary items and candies.

You may need to stock up on fats according to the regular ketogenic foods. Using that would speed up ketosis, as it is the physiological state that induces your body to burn stored fats rather than carbohydrates, eventually speeding up your weight reduction, nevertheless, because carbohydrates are just about anything and fats stored in different ways, which is not always healthy. People make mistakes here, especially in keto diets. Some of those mistakes are discussed here:

- **Jumping into the Keto diet too quickly.** You consume toast, burgers, and noodles one day, and you plan to start a ketogenic diet the next day. But you need to understand that your body needs time to adjust to new things. Cut down on carbs gradually, which will help your body get used to this new energy pathway.

- **Not drinking enough water.** You don't just have to be careful about what you eat. You need to make sure that you drink plenty of water throughout the day. The dramatic reduction in carbs' consumption on the keto diet will contribute to water and electrolyte imbalances. Carbohydrates are processed in your body with the help of water.

- **Not being aware of Keto challenges.** When your body enters ketosis, it makes major changes in your body. The whole energy pathway shifts from glucose to ketones. Because of these changes, you might notice signs of ketogenic flu. You might feel extremely tired or fatigued. You might also experience body pains or headaches. Sometimes people feel nauseous. If you aren't aware of these problems, you might feel like you are doing something wrong and might give up on a keto diet.

- **Not taking enough supplements.** It would help if you took multivitamins to keep your body in a healthy state. They boost your energy levels. It is advised to take calcium, potassium, zinc or magnesium supplements. Take omega-3 supplements too.

- **Not taking healthy fats.** Take fats from mussels, oysters or salmon etc. You can also use cod liver oil or extra virgin olive oil for it. Seeds like flax or chia seeds are also a good option. They are keto-friendly foods and store good cholesterol.

- **Not consulting any doctor.** Most keto diet supporters pursue it when they're trying to do it on a specific disorder. You should consult any doctor or nutritionist before starting any meal plan. Your doctor will be aware of your medical condition and will adjust your medicines according to it. They will also tell you if you should go for this diet or not.

- **Eating too little or too much.** Vegetables also have some amount of sugar in them. So it would help if you were careful about how much you are eating them. You might overeat carbs if you are not keeping track of it. Or on the other hand, you might be taking too little vegetables, which may cause constipation. Take care of your portions and count your carbs. Eat vegetables with less starch in them and are nutritious, such as cucumbers, broccoli, peppers, onions, asparagus and green veggies.

- **Not eating nutritious foods.** Some people worry too much about carbs, and they end up eating less than they need to. This makes them weak and causes many nutritional deficiencies. It feels as though keto's main purpose is to reduce carbohydrates dramatically, but it's not only that. It's good to cut on carbs but make sure that you take highly nutritious food to compensate for it. Take foods rich in omega-3. Snack on the whole and keto-friendly foods. Many licensed dietitians are not a fan of keto since nutritional problems may result from it. From itchy, dry skin to inadequate scar healing, many health problems can result in exhaustion, stress, and weight gain from inadequate nutrients intake.

- **You might not be measuring your macros properly.** For getting your desired results from the Keto diet, you need to track your macronutrients properly. Don't compare your count with anyone else's. Your requirement might be different from the one you might be comparing it with. If you reach a plateau with losing weight because you don't get the keto diet's maximum advantages, it could be either you are not getting enough fats or proteins, or you are not taking enough calories. Calculate the particular requirements for nutrients first. Then, see if you're on board with the directions below.

- **Taking so much stress.** Cortisol levels increase while you're depressed. And high levels of cortisol will disrupt the development of natural hormones and induce excessive weight gain. Stress makes adrenal glands produce more cortisol. It activates glucose accumulation in the body. Your blood sugar levels get disturbed. It also affects the functioning of insulin. Glucose keeps circulating in your body. High levels of blood sugar allow it more difficult for the body to generate and use ketone molecules.

- In comparison, constant stress will seriously discourage the development of hormones, which can induce cravings, sleep disorders, and even more significant hormonal problems. Following a low carb diet will bring a reasonably significant amount of stress on your body at the outset. So, once your body is adjusted to ketosis, you mustn't undergo any additional dietary adjustments.

- **Not making lifestyle adjustments.** Start working out along with the keto diet. Don't jump too quickly to hard exercises. Start gradually and progressively increase the time and number of exercises. Take enough sleep and on time one. Take part in leisure activities to stay motivated. It is important to have a healthy mind for a healthy body. Try meditation, mindfulness and yoga exercises. Try deep breathing exercises. For weight control, emotional clarity, and so much more, a keto diet is a successful strategy. But it requires a little more work to get the best results out of keto.

Chapter 5: How is Keto Diet different for Women over Fifty?

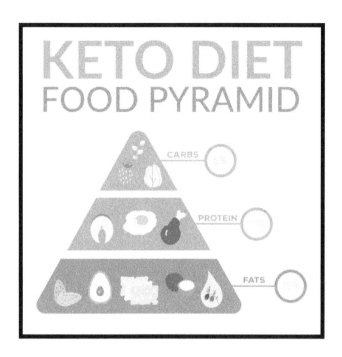

The outcome of any diet depends on a lot of factors. It depends on your metabolism rate, body structure, medical conditions and gender etc. This chapter will discuss how and why a keto diet is different for women.

5.1 Hormonal changes in Women

From fertility to tension to the body's metabolism rate, feminine hormones are linked to everything. Dependent on your menstruation cycles, the absence of proper sleep and consuming fewer carbs, the levels of these hormones even fluctuate. Men also have hormones, but women's hormones are more susceptible to fluctuations. As the ketogenic diet is a fairly radical transition for the human body to deal with, if you are not cautious, you will end up messing your hormones.

A decrease in Estrogen levels

Hormone levels change with age. As you grow older, estrogen levels decrease. Low levels of estrogen cause:

- Weaker bones

- Lower sex desire

- Dry vagina

- Poor sleep

- Mood swings

When women are above 40 or 45 years, they are most likely to experience menopause. At that time, their hormone levels are really high. The decrease in estrogen levels causes menopause. So a high- fat diet like a keto diet is preferred here and has shown good results.

Elevated Cortisol Levels

Cortisol is also known as a stress chemical, and it appears when there is not enough sugar in the bloodstream to relieve stress. This also disturbs insulin levels in the blood and makes it hard to lose weight.

Women every month have to contend with periods and experience those painful premenstrual syndrome symptoms. Cravings for candy becomes even more powerful, which makes it a struggle to remain in keto. Because you hang on to more fluids, you feel sluggish and weigh more. Consuming food is a severe challenge when you are so swollen, and discomfort tends to radiate down from your abdomen so that you may not even be hungry.

You will want to skip on meat and vegetables. You'll feel extremely tired and exhausted. You'll also have headaches, especially if you aren't taking enough water. It is important to balance your electrolytes with water. Cramps, cravings and mood swings make it hard to stick to the keto diet.

Effect of taking low carbs.

Although it is not suggested for men on the keto diet to consume too little carbohydrates, you certainly can't do this as a woman. The rapid drop in carbohydrates will push the body into the starvation phase, where the fat burning process becomes slow. Your body is responsive to what you eat to cling to all the calories you'll be taking. You won't be able to lose any weight in this way. Not only can this shock to the bloodstream induce hormones such as cortisol to

75

avoid losing weight, but you will also potentially start gaining weight in the process. Simply introducing little extra carbohydrates in your diet will give your emotions the positive signal that all is good, and it will start the weight loss phase by burning fat. You need to take more carbs if you are doing strenuous exercises or muscle building exercises.

Calorie Intake

A keto diet decreases your hunger, meaning you feel less hungry. Although it's awesome not to be on the lookout for food all the time, this advantage can lead you to forget to eat food. You might think it's great because you are taking few calories, but that's not healthy. Yes, we know to lose weight, you need to build a calorie shortage, but your body still needs enough calories to do several essential things. To healthily lose weight by taking balanced calories. If you are a woman and you are cutting on carbs, then you need to take more fats in your diet, especially if you are experiencing any of the following:

- Doing fat burning exercises.

- Breastfeeding.

- Having abnormal hormone levels.

- Metabolic problems.

5.3 Pregnancy and Breastfeeding

One of the most helpful strategies to boost the odds of pregnancy is to go for a keto diet. Most people discover that they have PCOS-induced fertility problems, which may trigger their ovaries to avoid ovulation and render conception very hard. This subject is discussed in more detail by our guidance on ketosis during the time of pregnancy, but here's a short rundown of what you need to do:

- Do not target, when pregnant, for weight reduction. To build essential sections of your body, your developing baby requires all the nutrition and calories available.

- Avoid fasting, so your baby would be starving for the foods it requires to thrive and evolve fully.

- Increase the consumption of carbohydrates because of the development of muscles and other vital internal components includes glucose.

- During breastfeeding, do not slash calories since it is what produces milk. The fewer calories you consume, you'll have less milk availability.

5.4 Meal preparation for Keto diet

If you have to cook and plan all the meals in your home, you will feel exhausted with making ketogenic and other food alternatives, particularly if you have kids. If you don't have support to plan all your meals and that for anyone else, this can easily make it hard to remain consistent with your keto diet. Plus, since women prefer to see mealtimes more like social events than refueling sessions. When everyone around you is eating their favorite meals and only eating keto foods, it might get hard for you to manage.

5.5 How to overcome these challenges

A keto diet does not have to be a disappointment for the body; it may be the best move for your wellbeing.

Gradually decrease consumption of carbs.

It's a bit easier for men to go for the keto diet, but it takes time to adjust to women. Start by monitoring your daily food consumption if you haven't begun a ketogenic diet yet. This can allow you the experience of weighing your diet and monitoring your keto macros. Let's presume that you are a normal woman who consumes 250 g of carbohydrates a day. While the fewer carbohydrates you consume can get through ketosis quicker, it doesn't require dramatic steps to find progress. They were found to experience substantial decreases in their blood sugar, insulin tolerance, cholesterol levels and testosterone levels. The gradual reduction in carbs would encourage your body to change and adapt with fewer carbs intake. If you feel sluggish, unable to complete your exercises, and always hungry, you will need to introduce a couple of extra carbohydrates to your day before you're used to fat.

Experiment with Intermittent Fasting

When you go hours without consuming any meals or snacks, intermittent fasting is where you fast for sixteen hours of the day and then eat within a particular eight-hour window. This type of fasting offers a rest from the tiresome work of food digestion for the body. Your body will focus on restoring itself and regulating the hormones throughout this period off, rather than going through the process of digestion. And you can use the fat stores for energy as your body completes all these things and becomes a little hungry, so you don't consume more calories than you are burning. Fasting lets you maintain ketosis quicker, meaning that you are losing weight fastly.

One research found that over eighty-four percent of participants had substantial weight reduction effects in only two months. Although supporting pure fat reduction, it still retains muscle mass. In another experiment, as subjects were separated into classes, they ate the same number of calories, but some used the fasting method, and others missed it. Researchers observed that intermittent fasting participants shed more weight, retained their muscle mass and got rid of pure fat. Since we realize the muscles improve the metabolism and burn further calories at rest, this is an excellent method. Research also suggests that intermittent fasting will decrease your:

- Risk of cardiac issues.

- Cholesterol levels.

- Body Inflammation.

And in one survey of many participants, scientists had women prolong their fasting hours overnight. They noticed that those who fasted for fewer than thirteen hours had a greater chance of breast cancer than those who fasted for thirteen hours or longer. Decreased sugar levels and good sleep were also found to be related to fasting.

After consuming a quick dinner before 7 to 8 pm, tucking in for a good night's rest and not having anything until you get up before you've reached the required fourteen-hour fasting date, the best way to get into intermittent fasting is. Because every night you can get at least 8 hours of sleep, by the time you wake up, you are already passed half of your fasting part. At this time, don't do endurance or extreme strengthening exercises, as you would most definitely flame out. Instead, consider meditation or going for walks.

Control your cravings on periods.

When it comes to period cravings, we're not all the same, but normally women dream of sugar, carbohydrates and fast food during this time of menstruation. Unfortunately, all these food cravings are really high in calories. But on keto, you cannot have sugary items or processed foods. So try to look for alternative food recipes.

- For sweet cravings, you can try having keto bars. You can make it by using dark chocolate, stevia etc. You can make keto chia pudding. You can make keto brownies or cookies as well.

- For salty food cravings, You can try making kale chips. You can have cauliflower with cheese. You can have zucchini noodles.

- And for your emotional wellbeing, stay away from the weighing scale before and after the week of your cycle. But strive not to skip the gym with cramps.

Introduce Conditioning for Resistance

Growing more muscles will improve your appetite, burn more calories at rest, and help your physique appear healthier while not losing much weight. So, work out for twenty to thirty minutes with heavyweights at least two times a week. This helps in losing weight and building strength.

5.6 Maintain a Keto Report of your food intake

To ensure you reach all of your macros, you may need to monitor your food consumption on the keto diet. To keep all these estimates coordinated, you may want to utilize a food monitoring software. Yet, it would help if you suggested maintaining a keto diary as well.

You should use this room to log how you feel in keto life because a woman's body is responsive to adjustments. You would be able to track stats and improvements like yours here:

- Body priorities
- Weight
- Body metrics
- Mood swings and thought
- Regeneration of exercise
- Food cravings

While you do not feel comfortable monitoring any of these items, it can be surprisingly useful for your physician or gynecologist over the long run. You would be able to spot trends or even food items that you don't handle well. And if you require more nutrients for your body, you'll have a clearer idea of which ones will improve the best.

Take Keto-friendly vitamins.

Cranberry juice used to treat female tract infections is high in sugar, so you should find its alternative supplement, which could have the same benefits. For healthier hair, nails, eyes, joints and metabolism, you should incorporate collagen into your diet. When you are just beginning keto or come off a cheat day, ketones will help you hit ketosis quicker so that they dominate the chart as one of the strongest cash keto supplements you can find. You'll be able to regain charge of your life and get started with all this knowledge.

5.7 How to Increase Estrogen levels on a Keto Diet

The best way to tell for sure is to have an expert's diagnosis if you're afraid that you have decreased estrogen levels. If you still haven't reached that step, you would want to know how to naturally raise estrogen levels when keeping on the keto diet. It could be possible for this guide to steer you in the correct direction. But first, it's crucial to realize why estrogen is essential for your wellbeing at any age and have the right amounts.

Functions of Estrogen Hormone

It is the most common and most thought about when it is about female hormone levels, but very few people recognize its functions. It is important to have a firm understanding of estrogen, how it evolves with time, and what you should do to maintain the estrogen levels in a stable range since it is necessary for your wellbeing. Ovaries and adrenal glands that produce sex hormones also produce it. In the puberty years, it induces the growth of the vagina and its structures. It also plays its role in developing breasts in females and makes women's pelvis broader than men. It also regulates the menstrual cycle in females. One of its main functions is to allow an egg to be released every month, and then it decreases rapidly after ovulation. It also induces the uterus and cervix to expand and become thick and develop mucous secretions for proper sexual operation during a woman's menstrual period. Over a woman's lifespan, hormone levels continuously shift and decrease dramatically. Estrogen plays a crucial function in cardiac wellbeing as well. It enhances stem cell viability by improving your lipid and cholesterol levels and reduces the risk of cardiac diseases. Your cardiac functioning can be placed at risk by low estrogen levels.

What happens to estrogen over the years?

After menopause, women tend to have lower estrogen levels and that's why the risk of heart and other diseases increases in them. Good estrogen levels have been shown to decrease the likelihood of diabetes and boost insulin activity. Insulin tolerance, which opens the door for other metabolic disorders, may be produced by a mild to extreme estrogen levels drop. Research shows that while stable before menopause in women has sufficient estrogen levels that shield them from metabolic disorders, insulin tolerance may be triggered by even a small reduction in estrogen levels. It also multiplied the risk of cancer, particularly in the cervix, ovaries, breasts etc. There could be a much greater chance of ovarian and breast cancer for women who have experienced menopause and estrogen deficiency. In females beyond the stage of producing children and are in menopause, estrogen is named estrone. The most popular estrogen source in women who aren't pregnant is released in the ovaries. That type of estrogen is called estradiol. Estriol is a lesser type of estrogen produced by a woman's placenta at the time of pregnancy and becomes more powerful while a woman is in that phase because her body's system no longer triggers the release of an egg every month. While women are more tend to encounter declines in estrogen after years of having children. Women that are also ovulating will feel reduced levels of estrogen as well.

How can you detect reduced estrogen levels?

There are some medical explanations why the levels of estrogen might be down. You might be going through menopause. If you have thyroid issues or any other congenital disease that might affect your estrogen levels. The working of endocrine glands also affects your hormone levels. Doing too much exercise or not taking enough calories and being weak can also have drastic effects on your hormone levels. If you notice any of the following signs, then it means your estrogen levels are low, and you need to consult a doctor:

- Irregular menstrual cycle

- Trouble sleeping or disturbed patterns

- Mood swings or irritability issues

- Anxiety or depression

- Fatigue or tiredness

- Lower sex drive

- Urinary tract infections

- Dry vagina

- Experiencing pain while having sex

- Tender breasts

It's necessary to recognize that this is not a good decision before you attempt to use them to diagnose by yourself the source of the symptoms. These signs can correlate with several other complications, including serious medical problems before you start addressing low estrogen levels on your own. You should consult a doctor. You could end up getting so many in your bloodstream if you want to raise your hormone levels while they are already where they should be. If you think anything is abnormal, get checked because your doctor will have an updated image of your estrogen levels stand before you initiate some medication. And these recommendations could be the perfect complement to your gyne's plan for those of you who have a reported low estrogen level.

How to Improve Estrogen Levels

It would help if you also take some tips to raise your hormone levels, along with the medication choices the doctor has scheduled.

Consume soy-rich foods

Estrogens are found in soy products. These ingredients would not raise the levels of estrogen. It is where the plan for the doctor falls in. As far as beans and soy milk are concerned, they are rich in carbohydrates, so they didn't enter the list. Although you can not get estrogen directly from the foods you consume, you can have on phytoestrogens-packed foods, such as:

- Flaxseeds

- Vegetables like cauliflower, sprouts, kale and broccoli etc.

- Sesame seeds

- Seeds of Pumpkin

- Hazelnuts, pistachios, walnuts.

You shouldn't have any problem incorporating these into your diet because these ingredients are nutritious and keto-friendly. The consistency of the food is therefore important for healthy levels of estrogen. The avoidance of refined, processed foods and sugary items helps maintain proper processing of your body and provides all it requires to generate adequate estrogen.

Sugar Consumption

It has been found that sugar had enough strength to completely stop estrogen production in one analysis. The analysis revealed that all types of sugar had this decreasing estrogen effect. Especially the type found in fruits and vegetables as well as refined foods. For those adopting a keto diet, fructose is still poor since consuming a lot of sugar can knock you out of ketosis. On the other side, you may be delighted to hear that having coffee once a day is a positive thing, but just in certain cases.

Caffeine Intake

Researchers discovered a significant correlation between caffeine consumption and estrogen levels in females. Asian people boosted their levels of estrogen by consuming coffee twice a day. At the same time, white females lowered their levels of estrogen. Black women boosted their levels of estrogen, yet to be deemed important, it was not enough. One correlation researchers found is that caffeine can worsen symptoms of menopause. Consuming a lot of caffeine will often bring the body into tension, which further produces cortisol, affecting the general hormonal equilibrium. A faster start of menopause can often result from consuming so much caffeine. If you are still low on estrogen and Caucasian, it might not be wise to go above the 200 mg caffeine per day. Alternatively, restrict yourself to consuming one improved coffee a day. It will help to raise your vitality, weight control, metabolism and decrease inflammation.

Exercise regularly

Don't do too much workout but make exercising regularly a habit. Working too hard or too vigorously will induce more hormones such as cortisol to be secreted by the body. Your whole hormone equilibrium can be thrown off when this occurs. Working out can always be a good option, but for as much as three to five days per week, you'll want to maintain the strength at a moderate pace. One of the points that exercise is advantageous is that it will avoid the buildup of fat that continues to arise in women after reaching menopause due to the decrease in estrogen levels.

Quit Smoking

You do realize that active and passive smoking is terrible for your well being. Studies have found active and passive smoke to lower hormone levels in both males and females, among other health risks. And since estrogen helps hold calcium in bones, there is also an increased risk of osteoporosis for those who smoke, particularly menopausal women. Quit smoking and concentrate on your wellbeing.

Use Herbal Teas

You can also try herbal teas or other supplements for improving your estrogen levels. Chasteberry is a tea that may alleviate tenderness or discomfort in breasts and other menstrual problems typically seen in Asia. And one study noticed that this tea could improve vaginal secretions, especially in menopausal women, but further research is required to validate this.

Dong Quai, a popular tea, has been used to alleviate hot sweats, facilitate menopausal adjustment, and reduce premenstrual syndrome symptoms.Tea Red clover is filled with estrogens, which implies that it might boost and stabilize decreased estrogen levels when drunk as a tea. Suppose you have been diagnosed with decreased levels of estrogen. In that case, it is always a safe idea to contact the doctor to decide if the recovery strategy will include the methods in this book. You would easily practice these tips to boost the estrogen levels on a ketogenic diet.

Chapter 6: The Ultimate Keto Guide for Older Women

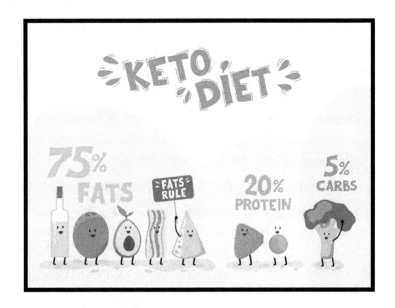

You might have seen and heard a lot about the famous keto diet. By using the keto diet, you healthily lose weight by eating in portions and avoiding carbs. If you want to go for a keto diet, you should know what you are going for.

6.1 Keto Diet Expectations

Your expectations for the keto diet should be realistic. This chapter explains what you'll get to experience in the starting days of the keto diet and how to deal with them.

Ketosis

The ketogenic diet, which promotes consuming food high in fats, adequate proteins and low in carbs. This is necessary for the body to achieve Ketosis, the natural source of nutrition, or a condition where fat starts burning for energy production. The ketosis phase starts in one or two days. Your body starts using ketones for producing energy instead of glucose. People might think that they only have to avoid sugary foods or fatty foods to enter ketosis, but they need to cut on carbs in reality. You have to cut on berries, starchy vegetables, dairy foods and legumes etc. Monitor your carbs intake and don't exceed the specified amount of calories.

Lack of motivation in start

As keto is a highly restrictive diet, it won't be easy to stay consistent. It would help if you were motivated and determined. You might experience ketogenic flu in the starting days of ketosis. In it, you will feel extreme tiredness and fatigue. You might want to give up on it. You might face headaches or body aches. Your body needs time to adjust to new energy pathways because shifting from glucose to ketones is a big change. So in the start, you might feel a lack of energy in your body.

Workout Routine

When muscles don't get the glucose or carbs they used to get before the keto diet, they get tired and exhausted. Because of this, you will not feel like working out. Your stamina and power will be reduced, and you will have to push yourself to workout daily. You should do light-intensity exercises even if you don't feel like working out.

Experiencing side effects

You might face gut issues when you go on the keto diet. Your body's digestion system needs time to adjust to a new routine, so your gut health might be compromised at the start because of the lack of consumption of fiber. You might have problems like nausea, abdominal pain, diarrhea or vomiting. So make sure that you get enough fiber in your diet. Consume vegetables like greens, avocado and broccoli etc. Drink plenty of water. Take multivitamins and other supplements to keep yourself healthy.

Diversity

Everyone is different and they have different body mechanisms. Everyone's metabolism works in different and unique ways. You cannot compare yourself or your results with anyone else. This only leads to depression and a lack of motivation. Someone might lose weight in days and some might shed the same number of pounds in months. Results depend on how consistently you follow your diet. Losing weight doesn't only depend on fixing your diet. It also depends on your lifestyle, physical activity and stress management. Stay positive and appreciate yourself for trying to stick to a healthier lifestyle. Consult a nutritionist.

Water consumption

Drink plenty of water to avoid the side effects of the keto diet. Water removes all the wasteful products and doesn't let them store in your body. In ketosis, it is important to keep a balance between water and electrolytes concentration. Make sure you don't get dehydrated.

Take enough calories

You might not feel like eating anything at the start. But don't deprive your body of the essential nutrients. Take enough calories according to your body requirements. The Keto diet doesn't starve you. You have to eat lots of fat and fewer carbs. People will find it difficult to take fats at the start, but you'll get used to it with time.

Lifestyle Adjustments

The keto diet not only requires dietary changes but also needs lifestyle changes. You have to find and adopt an effective, healthy and stable plan that will help you lose weight, get benefits and stick to the ketogenic diet. Take time to discover what foods and ways suit your body and then stick to them. You can also consult a nutritionist to help you with it.

Keto Diet Results

You should know what you'll get at the end of your keto diet journey. This helps you in staying motivated. By following a keto diet, you can expect the following results:

- It helps in losing weight.

- It improves your cardiovascular health.

- It improves your brain health and functioning.

- It makes your skin condition better.

- It improves your metabolic disorders.

- It is helpful for diabetic and hypertensive patients.

- It helps to treat PCOS.

- It helps in balancing hormone levels and endocrine health.

•

Who shouldn't go for a Keto Diet?

If you have liver issues, you shouldn't go for a high-fat diet like the keto one. If you cannot stay consistent with it because it is a highly restrictive diet, don't even start it. If you have the following health problems, then don't go for a ketogenic diet:

- Kidney problems

- Pancreatitis

- Type-1 diabetes

- Pregnant or nursing women

- Chronic and serious medical issues

Short terms Effects of the Keto Diet

- Going into ketosis in one to two days.

- Ketogenic flu for a week.

- Tiredness and fatigue

- Mood swings

- Gut problems

Long terms effects of the Keto Diet

- Weight loss

- Improved cardiovascular health

- Improved hormone levels

- Improved insulin regulation

- Improved self-esteem

- Improved skin

- Detoxified body

6.2 Myths about the Keto Diet and their Clarification

Myths about ketosis and acidosis

Ketosis is what induces the keto to burn fat. You get through it while you go on a keto diet, a physiological condition where the body uses fat food for energy sources. The body breaks down, burns fat and turns it into ketone bodies during this process. This is not the same thing as acidosis, a possibly dangerous condition that develops when the body doesn't get enough insulin and the amount of ketone molecules is elevated.

Myths about weight gain or loss

Keto enables you to lose weight healthily. You can also switch off from it for some time, but you'll get results whenever you go back to it. It would only bring you back to losing all the weight. People mostly don't educate themselves about the keto diet and jump into it without realizing what they are getting into. Thus, they cheat on it more than often, which gets them out of ketosis, and they don't get any results.

Myths about calorie intake

As everybody has different body metabolisms, so they also have different calorie requirements. Some people need fewer calories, while some people need more calories. It all depends on your medical condition, body weight, body mechanism and other factors. Some people have genetic conditions and cannot use high-fat foods, making it difficult for them to follow a keto diet.

Myths about food choices in a keto diet

In this diet, you are asked to give up on high-carb-containing foods and eat healthier fat foods. You cannot eat sugary or processed foods. You can only consume berries and low-sugar fruits. You can consume low starch vegetables only. Don't eat saturated fats. Go for unsaturated ones. Take high fiber foods. Take unprocessed and fresh foods that have vitamins, minerals and all the essential nutrients. You can have the following items:

- Zucchini

- Broccoli

- Cucumbers

- Tomatoes

- Cauliflower

- Berries like strawberries, blueberries etc.

- Eggs

- Meat

- Fish

Take proteins in moderation or else they will increase glucose levels in the blood and stop ketosis. Moreover, too many proteins make too many amino acids and increase ketone molecules in the body, which is quite harmful.

6.3 How can you stick to low carb for a long time?

Bear in mind that the body adapts to burning fat for food, not carbohydrates, and takes a couple of days. As you realize the cravings go down, this will motivate you to battle the candy ghost. It's sometimes out of a foolish attempt to give in to sweet cravings, often because of hunger, tension or tiredness, and you'll accept that you're generally left saying it wasn't worth it anyway. Know that you will have sugar and carb cravings for a few days, and you are powerful enough to resolve them. Typically, eating anything will aid as cravings strike, but cheese, vegetables, olives, boiled egg, etc., are all safe choices. When you're starving, don't go hungry, have the correct option and make sure your refrigerator/cupboards are filled with low-carb foods. Only imagine, you could be adapted to burning fat in three or four days and well on your way to a healthy you!

Don't depend on exercising so much. Although exercise is perfect for its cardiovascular advantages, the secret to success is what you consume. So don't reward yourself with a high-carb meal after a workout. Pick yourself right back up and get back on track if you have a moment of vulnerability. One hack would not derail all your attempts. However, slipping into the pit of absolutely having this causes you to lose the story's will. Choose whether to be measured or not. Remember that the device tests body fat and absorb water weight, skin, bone, food and drink, which will fluctuate based on hormones, whether you have consumed, whether you have exercised, etc. Identify and don't purchase the things you can't resist. You can't consume what's not there. Know, though, that it requires time to transition to burning fat for energy so that you have the patience to keep moving! Many people who have been good in the long run would tell you that they have gone through times of little results but have kept solid, and it was worth it.

Before you can go to the restaurant or bar, the easiest way to do it is to glance at the menu online. Get a good picture of the low-carb option you create in your head, and don't deviate. Note that you should consume loads of lovely low-carb recipes. Eat fat from oils, fish, butter, veggies, cream, avocados, etc. The fat can lead you quality and making meals taste fantastic too. Carbohydrates are part of a nutritious meal schedule because many greens are included from day one. If you are hungry, continue to eat between meals or raise the portion size marginally.

6.4 Important Reminders about the Keto Diet

We have an idea that it's not straightforward to get started- you to develop many different routines, find time to prepare your meals and cook and exercise. Don't get overwhelmed at the start. It'll demotivate you, and you might give up. You ought to have a good understanding of why you choose to alter your eating patterns before you undertake a low-carbohydrate diet and remember what made you select that specific diet. One of the strongest solutions out there is low-carb and keto, giving a start anytime you set a new target, both for losing weight and overall wellness. These diets help you control your hunger, balance your sugar levels and insulin regulation, and have shown to be very successful. And a host of other opportunities for wellbeing.

You ought to make a strategy and stick to that if you wish to excel in something. Getting a ketogenic diet provides you with straightforward instructions to achieve that target. With every day, you would know precisely what to consume and how to get those macros. You need to complete that targeted calorie intake.

Low carbohydrate and ketogenic are also a type of clean eating and making lifestyle changes. It is not an easy diet that you should perform and then discontinue in about some weeks. You ought to adjust your entire way of living to shed those extra pounds and effectively hold it off. Old patterns are what brought you there and the outcome would be the same if you start eating junk food again. A sedentary lifestyle and unhealthy eating will take you back and you'll have to start from zero again. After you're through the weight reduction journey, you may want to turn to another diet that lets you remain where you want to try another diet. The key point is, you have to be conscious of your dietary intake and nutrient requirements. There are lots of fantastic choices.

You haven't gained weight in two weeks, but you won't also drop weight in two weeks. Make targets that are practical and strive on them. Within the first few days of Ketosis, certain people may lose many pounds. However, it is realistic to lose some pounds in a month or two, and most individuals will do it by remaining disciplined and keeping to their macros. If you have something to lose, your improvement will be smoother initially, so the closer you get to your target weight, the harder it would be and your body will resist change. You would generally see a fast weight reduction in the first few days or weeks as you first implement a ketogenic or a low-carbohydrate diet, but much of it is water weight. You may be inclined to create a massive deficiency and diet as fast as you can, but that's not a good plan, and you may end up getting disappointed.

Although others tend to create a brief and excruciating calorie reduction to rapidly remove the extra weight and finish with it, only a few succeed with such a plan. Two to three weeks after beginning them, many individuals give up on these diets. They just get bored of consuming too little carbs. If you lose weight quite soon, holding the weight off later will not be easy as you will be vulnerable to bouts of great appetite if you go back to consuming tonnes of carbohydrates, particularly. It might be because your body doesn't want to adjust, and it will fight weight loss. It would be less painful for you if you're moving slowly, and you have a lot greater chance of keeping your fresh, new weight for the long term.

Even though the keto diet is the critical aspect of weight loss, keeping healthy can probably not harm you. To thrive, you don't need to perform countless hours of doing cardio- in reality, and this could be harmful since it might raise your appetite and render your food more challenging to handle. Low-intensity exercises, strength lifting, or other workouts may be amazing options to sustain a greater deficit and gain muscle mass. Both of these may be paired with a ketogenic or a low-carbohydrate diet effectively.

It is also good to travel around during regular tasks since it will improve your health. Your thermogenic system appears to get smaller while you're on a diet, which is the body's action not to shed the weight you're attempting to get rid of, but you ought to make a deliberate effort to prevent it. Your results will be affected in the first few weeks of the ketogenic diet because your body needs time to adjust. Keep driving, and you're not going to miss it.

Dieting typically indicates that you can feel certain harmful or undesired effects with time, such as increased appetite. Ketogenic and low-carbohydrates are considered to better regulate your appetite, although it doesn't guarantee you're never going to be hungry. Have low-carb snacks when you feel hungry or drink plenty of water. Typically, the ketogenic flu and adaptation process is not enjoyable either, but they will soon be done. The ketogenic flu persists only a few days in most situations. Although the tolerance to fat requires around four to six weeks, they are easy to handle.

Life will make this process hard if you don't identify your goals. Let your close ones realize that you are moving on to a new target and ask for guidance and motivation from them. Bear in mind even if you are a working mom who fails to make time for your body, your wellbeing is highly essential to your loved one's wellbeing.

The Keto diet doesn't have to be costly, though, because you can always make things fit while you're on a small budget. And try to remember, being obese is far riskier than making a few changes today. There are lots of free tools here; utilize them. At the start, both ketogenic and low-carbohydrate diets may be difficult to stick to. It's nice to have your close ones love you, but it may also be really important to find a group that will recognize your challenges and successes and remains accountable. Don't depend on inspiration and willpower, and these can carry you so far. Create a schedule instead, and adhere to it.

Make sure you remain below the carbohydrate quota, prepare your foods before time. This makes ketogenic and low-carbohydrate diets even easier to carry your food to function. Design the drills. If you need some, prepare your treats. Don't feed out of hunger or stress, and if you're very hungry, have a keto snack. You can also arrange time in your calendar to prepare and work out so that you don't have to focus on inspiration to do it. You will still go far more than a mere determination by creating good behaviors. We're routine beings and love peace. In the long term, creating fresh, healthier routines can be really good for you. Make the following things your new habits:

- Tracking macros

- Taking stairs

- Going on walks

- Meal prepping

- Monitor calorie intake

- Drinking lots of water

- Doing exercise

- Avoiding sugary or processed items

In the start, it requires patience and determination, but as you get accustomed to it, it becomes a part of your life.

Don't make everything difficult when you go for a ketogenic way of living. Whenever you start feeling bored, please stick to the fundamentals and adjust it a bit.

- Focus on whole foods.

- Select a protein source.

- Incorporate fat when frying.

- Eat low-carb and non-starchy vegetables.

- Stick to a deficit of calories.

- Stay hydrated and maintain control of your electrolytes.

Remove all the high-carbohydrate stuff that may be tempting. Not consuming food that you don't have at your place is much better than making a deliberate attempt to avoid eating it. If you live around someone who doesn't adopt a low-carbohydrate lifestyle, encourage them to support you by keeping their food separately from yours. An integral feature in both ketogenic and low-carbohydrate diets is monitoring the macros. Carbohydrates are in every food out there and if you're not watching it, you might go over the carb quota without really being conscious of it. However, monitoring is not just about carbohydrates. Equally significant are the other macros. Protein is needed to preserve your muscles and other organs. Fat is needed to fulfill your energy requirements. It's important to weigh something with a scale while monitoring. And bear in mind that you can weigh the protein sources and vegetables fresh.

Conclusion

Keto diets are low in carbs, moderate in protein intake and high in fat consumption. This type of food intake helps your body in burning fat and losing weight. The human body is completely capable of running on ketones and many experiments demonstrate that this is the preferred fuel for the heart muscles, especially the brain cells. In this diet, you keep track of your macros, calorie intake and lose weight healthily. Women's health is very sensitive and reacts to changes in diet, lifestyle or stress etc. It is important to keep everything in mind before starting this diet. This book explains how you can benefit from this diet and why you should go for it. All the pros and cons are described briefly in this book. It improves your sleep pattern and mental health. It helps in maintaining your sugar levels and insulin regulation. It improves endocrine health, and that's why it is important in women. Women's hormones fluctuate and react rapidly to such changes. It also improves skin condition. It helps you to lose weight without starving yourself. It is a restrictive diet, but it is a healthier one. It might be difficult for you to get used to it, but you'll eventually. The removal of different food groups can render it challenging to adhere to. An individual absorbs much of the calories from proteins and fats in this diet rather than from carbohydrates. In the keto diet, ketones are used to start producing energy. This program stresses the elimination of fat rather than a keto diet for nutritional benefits. Food options for each category are also explained in this book. People often use a keto diet to lose weight, but it may help cure some heart problems, neurological problems, seizures, PCOS, etc. It is important to make lifestyle changes and dietary changes; its detail and method are also explained in this book. This book is a complete guide for women over fifty to start a keto diet. It will help in improving their health and will also increase their life span. In persons that reduce their carbohydrate consumption, you usually see improved outcomes. For the first few months of a ketogenic diet, hold the carbohydrates as minimal as possible. Keep things strict by absolutely leaving away unnecessary sugar and chemical sweeteners. Taking them out cuts sugar cravings significantly. Dehydration or loss of electrolytes causes the most common issues. Ensure you consume lots of water, salt your meals, and take a multivitamin before beginning keto (and also in the long run). You should request electrolyte supplements separately if you're still having problems. Over-consumption of carbohydrates is too simple because they're in about everything that you usually eat. Keeping note of what you consume allows you to monitor and hold yourself responsible for your carb consumption. Do consult your doctor before going for this diet as it has its pros and cons. This book tries to aware of all the upcoming challenges that come with keto diets.

Keto Diet for Women

The Easiest Way to Lose Weight Quickly
including Delicious Recipesfor Increase
your energy and Start Your New Life
Immeditely

By Jason Smith

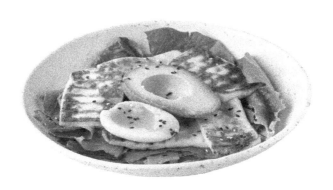

The trademarks that are used are without any consent, and the publication of the trademark is without permission or backing by the trademark owner. All trademarks and brands within this book are for clarifying purposes only and are the owned by the owners themselves s, not affiliated with this document.

Introduction

In today's time, the keto diet needs no introduction because of its many health benefit. A low carb, high-fat diet and weight loss aspect make it beneficial for all, especially women over 50. Ketogenic diets, or just "keto," have been popular for a long time. Conceptualized in the 1920s as an epilepsy cure, they presented the Atkins diet plan research, which became famous in the 1970s for the first time. Keto is back now. As with old age, people are more susceptible to more diseases like diabetes, Alzheimer's, epilepsy, cancer, obesity, which is the leading cause of all diseases. Keto provides many health benefits to combat these diseases. A very low carb, high-fat diet, which has several aspects with the low carb plan. It requires significantly lowering and replacing the consumption of carbohydrates with fat. This carbohydrate reduction places a body in a metabolic condition called ketosis. The body makes it extremely easy for itself to burn fat for energy as this process occurs. In the liver, it also converts fat into ketones, which can provide the brain with energy. Major declines in insulin levels and blood sugar may be induced by ketogenic diets that benefit people with diabetes. It has certain health benefits, along with elevated ketones. These habits are similar to successful weight reduction programs that have a shared strategy, the ultimate health for elder adults.

If someone has diabetes, they must consult their doctor first before switching to the keto diet suddenly and make gradual changes rather than sudden changes.

Chapter1:What is the keto diet

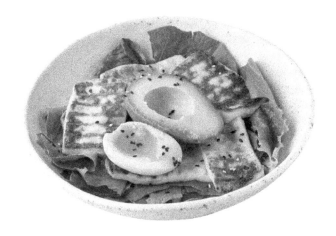

The low-carb, moderate protein, a higher-fat diet that can help you lose fat more efficiently is a keto or ketogenic diet. As shown in over 50 studies, it has many advantages for weight loss, fitness, and efficiency. That's why a rising number of physicians and healthcare practitioners suggest it. A keto diet is particularly useful for losing excess body fat, reducing appetite, and enhancing type 2 diabetes or metabolic syndrome. You cut most of the carbohydrates, such as sugar, soda, pastries, and white bread, that are easy to digest. In certain ways, it's similar to other low-carb diets.

When on a keto diet, you consume far fewer carbohydrates, retain moderate protein consumption, and increase your fat intake. The drop-in carb intake puts your body in a metabolic state called ketosis, where fat is burned for energy from your food and your body. If you consume less than 50 grams of carbohydrates a day, the body can gradually run out of fuel (blood sugar) that you can use easily. Usually, this takes 3 to 4 days. Then you're going to start breaking down fat and protein for energy, which can help you lose weight. It's called ketosis here. It is important to remember that a short-term diet is a ketogenic diet that focuses on weight loss rather than health benefits.

A "keto" or "ketogenic" diet is so named because it allows the body to generate tiny molecules of fuel called "ketones." It is an alternative fuel source for your body that can be used when there is a lack of blood sugar (glucose). Your liver creates ketones from fat when you eat very few carbs or very few calories. These ketones, especially for the brain, then serve as a fuel source throughout the body. The brain is a hungry organ that absorbs a lot of energy regularly and can't run directly on fat. It can only function on ketones or glucose. Your whole body changes its fuel source to run mostly on fat on a ketogenic diet, burning fat all day long. Fat burning will increase drastically when insulin levels fall very low. To burn them off, it becomes simpler to reach your fat stores.

It is perfect if you're trying to lose weight, but without the sugar peaks and valleys that often arise when eating high-carb meals, there can also be other benefits, such as less appetite and a constant supply of energy. It will help keep you focused and alert.

1.1 What does ketosis mean?

The body enters a metabolic state called ketosis as it releases ketones. Fasting-not eating anything-is the quickest way to get there, but no one can reliably fast forever, particularly not women over 50. Instead of carbohydrates, ketosis is a metabolic condition in which the body uses fat for food.

It happens when you decrease the intake of carbohydrates substantially, decreasing the body's supply of glucose (sugar), which is the main Source of energy for cells.

The most successful way of going into ketosis is to adopt a ketogenic diet. It typically includes reducing carb intake to about 20 to 50 grams a day and filling up on fats, fish, eggs, nuts, and healthy oils.

Moderating your intake of protein is also significant. If ingested in high quantities, protein may be transformed into glucose, delaying the transformation into ketosis.

You may also get into ketosis quicker by doing intermittent fasting. There are many different intermittent fasting ways, but the most common approach includes restricting food consumption to around 8 hours a day and the remaining 16 hours of fasting. There are available blood, urine, and breath tests that can help assess if you have reached ketosis by testing your body releases' number of ketones.

Some symptoms can also suggest that ketosis has occurred, including increased thirst, dry mouth, frequent urination, and reduced appetite or hunger.

Ketosis is a metabolic condition in which the body uses fat and ketones as the main fuel source rather than glucose (sugar).

In your liver, glucose is stored and released as required for energy. However, these glucose reserves become exhausted after carb intake has been exceptionally low for one to two days.

Via a process known as gluconeogenesis, your liver can make some glucose from amino acids in the protein you eat, but not nearly enough to fulfill all your brain's needs, which requires a constant supply of fuel.

Luckily, ketosis can provide an alternative source of energy for you, and especially for your brain.

In ketosis, ketones are formed at an accelerated rate by your body. Ketones, or ketone bodies, are made from the fat you eat in your liver and your fat in your body. Beta-hydroxybutyrate (BHB)acetoacetate and acetone are the three ketone bodies. In ketosis, ketones are formed at an accelerated rate by your body. Ketones, or ketone bodies, are made from the fat you eat in your liver and your fat in your body. Even while eating a higher-carb diet, the liver develops ketones regularly. It occurs mostly overnight as you sleep, but only in small quantities. When the levels of glucose and insulin decline, such as on a carb-restricted diet, the liver ramps up ketone output to supply the brain with energy.

When a certain threshold is reached for the number of ketones in your blood, you are known to have dietary ketosis. According to leading ketogenic diet experts, the requirement for nutritional ketosis is at least 0.5 mmol/L of BHBB, Dr. Steve Phinney and Dr. Jeff Volek (the ketone body measured in the blood). While you will achieve ketosis with both fasting and a keto diet, only a keto diet is sustainable over long periods. It seems to be a safe way of eating that individuals can follow indefinitely.

1.2 Do you need carbs for your brain to survive?

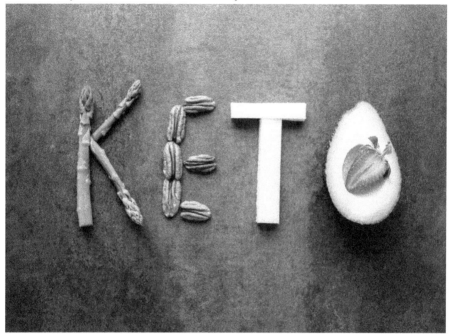

There's a long-standing and unfounded idea that the proper operation of the brain includes carbs. If you ask any dietitians how many carbs you should consume, they are likely to reply that to ensure your brain has a steady glucose supply; you need a minimum of 130 grams per day. It isn't the case, though. Even if you consume no carbohydrates at all, your brain will stay balanced and efficient. While it is true that your brain has high energy requirements and needs some glucose, there are plenty of ketones to provide a good portion of its power while you're in ketosis.

Fortunately, your liver will still generate the small amount of glucose your brain requires even under complete malnutrition conditions. This method allowed our hunter-gatherer ancestors to go without eating for long periods because they had access at all times to a fuel source: stored body fat. There are no adverse effects on brain activity from being in ketosis. On the contrary, when they are in ketosis, many individuals have indicated that they feel more mentally sharp.

1.3 Difference Vs. Ketoacidosis Between Dietary Ketosis

The definitions of ketosis and ketoacidosis are both distinct, but they sound similar. A type of 1 D.M. complication, the term 'ketoacidosis' refers to diabetic ketoacidosis (DKA). It is an extremely life-threatening illness that leads to ketones and blood glucose levels becoming dangerously elevated. Production takes place in ketosis and ketoacidosis, as well as in ketones. Ketosis is considered to be usually stable, while ketoacidosis can be life-threatening.

This mixture makes the blood highly acidic, directly targeting the functioning of sensory organs in the body, such as the liver and kidneys. It is of the utmost importance if this is the case that it is treated. With DKA, it can occur very rapidly. It can grow in just 24 hours. It is most prevalent among those with Type 1 diabetes whose bodies lack insulin. DKA, which is similar to sickness, inadequate diet, or not taking the right insulin dosage, may be responsible for several things. Many people with type 2 diabetes with little to no insulin production in the body are at risk of developing DKA.

Ketosis is a metabolic process that begins when the body is on a low diet of carbohydrates. The liver produces ketone bodies after this. The ketone body level rises to 8 mmol/l in ketosis without causing changes to the pH value. During ketoacidosis, ketone bodies' level is forced to increase to 20 mmol/l, resulting in decreased P.H. levels. Therefore, both ketoacidosis and ketosis contain ketones but have distinct efficacy.

Nutritional ketosis and diabetic ketoacidosis are disorders that are entirely different. Ketoacidosis is a medical emergency, while nutritional ketosis is safe and beneficial for health.

Sadly, the distinction between the two is not recognized by many health care practitioners.

If they don't take insulin, ketoacidosis occurs primarily in people with type 1 diabetes. Blood sugar and ketones rise to dangerous levels during diabetic ketoacidosis (DKA), disrupting the blood's delicate acid-base balance. BHB levels usually remain below five mmol/L for nutritional ketosis. However, people with diabetic ketoacidosis frequently have levels of BHB at or above ten mmol/L that are directly linked to their failure to produce insulin.

This graph illustrates the vast difference between ketosis and ketoacidosis in the number of ketones in the blood:

Many with type 2 diabetes who take drugs known as SGLT2 inhibitors, such as Invokana, Farxiga, or Jardiance, are other individuals who may get ketoacidosis.

Women who do not have diabetes can also, in rare cases, experience ketoacidosis while breastfeeding.

However, it is almost rare for most individuals capable of processing insulin to go into ketoacidosis.

1.4 What are ketones' bodies?

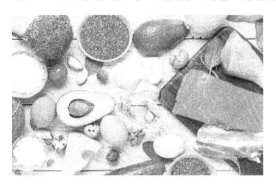

When there is an insulin deficiency in the blood, the body releases distinct chemicals. As an energy supplier, internal fat is often allowed to break down instead of using glucose (sugar). Acetone, acetoacetate, and beta-hydroxybutyrate are all ketone species that are considered toxic acid chemicals. Via the blood and into the urine, they pass. An additional way for the body to get rid of acetone in the lungs (respiration). Ketosis is when ketone bodies are present in the blood, and ketonuria is the urine that includes ketone bodies.

The liver ketone production house will produce ketone molecules at around 185 gs per day. Acetoacetate is a sub-form of liver-assembled ketones, while the predominant blood circulating ketone molecules is beta-hydroxybutyrate. These are combined with acetyl coenzyme A (CoA) after their formation and join the 'Krebs cycle.' Krebs' cycle is considered a part of the metabolic pathway that uses oxygen to burn fuel to produce energy in organisms' breathing.

It is where energy molecules are generated using them.

1.5 How to Get Started with Ketosis

There are two approaches that most followers refer to intermittent fasting or adopting a keto diet. To one degree or another, many proponents of ketosis combine the two approaches.

By restricting one's food consumption to a daily window (usually around eight hours) or incorporating a few very-low-calorie days into each week to drive the body into ketosis, intermittent fasting attempts to replicate the symptoms of a temporary famine.

On the other hand, consuming mostly fat plus a small amount of protein (because protein can be converted to glucose) and virtually nothing else means adopting a keto diet. Stephen Cunnane, a professor at the Research Centre on Aging at the University of Sherbrooke in Quebec, says, "The keto diet is designed to mimic the effect of fasting without actually starving." "Broadly speaking, they are doing the same."

But that isn't fast. By consuming less than around 50 grams of carbohydrates a day, we can only get into ketosis around a cooked pasta cup.

A ketogenic diet can be perfect for people who:

• Overweight is

• Having diabetes

They aim to improve their metabolic well-being.

It might be less appropriate for elite athletes or those wishing to add significant muscle or weight quantities.

It may also not be sustainable for the lifestyles and desires of certain individuals. Speak to your doctor about your diet routine and your objectives to determine whether you want a keto eating plan.

1.6 Keto diet styles

Several variations of the ketogenic diet exist, including:

A very low carb, moderate protein, and high-fat diet is the normal ketogenic diet (SKD). Usually, it contains 70% fat, 20% protein, and just 10% carbs (9Trusted Source).

A cyclical ketogenic diet (CKD): This diet requires higher carb refill times, such as five ketogenic days followed by two high carb days.

The targeted ketogenic diet (TKD): This diet makes it possible to add carbohydrates to workouts.

High protein ketogenic diet: It contains more protein than a regular ketogenic diet. Sometimes, the ratio is 60% fat, 35% protein, and 5% carbs.

Only the normal and high protein ketogenic diets have been extensively studied, however. More complex approaches are cyclical or targeted ketogenic diets, mainly used by bodybuilders or athletes.

For the most part, this book material refers to the traditional ketogenic diet (SKD), although the other variations still apply several of the same concepts.

People sometimes ask me about the various ways in which people can practice keto, and here are some of the most common:

KETO STRICT

- Controlling calories and macros strictly, usually with a control app
- Eating just safe, whole foods, concentrating on nutrients.
- Many carbs derive from low-carb vegetables.
- Even if total carb counts are poor, avoid wheat, gluten, artificial sweeteners, and added sugars.

LAZY KETO Just

- Track net carbs only OR eat keto foods without monitoring.
- The approach to food may or may not be clean (like strict keto) (like dirty keto)

DIRTY KETO

- An approach to keto "if it fits your macros."
- Controlling calories and macros strictly, usually with a control app
- Even if it is processed, artificial, or even sugar added, you can eat something as long as it suits your macros.
- Find out more here about Dirty Keto.

CARB Poor

- Similar to lazy, but more lenient on carbohydrates
- The carbon limit can be as high as 50 grams or even up to 100 grams for those who want more versatility.
- Moderate carb foods may also be allowed, in addition to keto-friendly foods,

Chapter 2: Body Symptoms of Ketosis

Your body gets into ketosis after you follow the diet for a few days, which means it has begun to use fat for energy. Diet newbies find it useful to monitor whether they're with a urine ketone strip or a blood-prick meter in ketosis. You'll finally understand what ketosis feels like and know if you're in it. This low-carb, high-fat diet can increase blood ketone levels when followed correctly. These provide your cells with a fresh fuel source and produce most of this diet's specific health benefits. Your body undergoes multiple biological changes on a ketogenic diet, including a drop in insulin levels and increased fat breakdown. When this occurs, your liver begins to generate large amounts of ketones to provide your brain with energy. It can also be difficult to recognize, however, whether you're in ketosis or not. Here are ten normal, both positive and negative, signs and symptoms of ketosis.

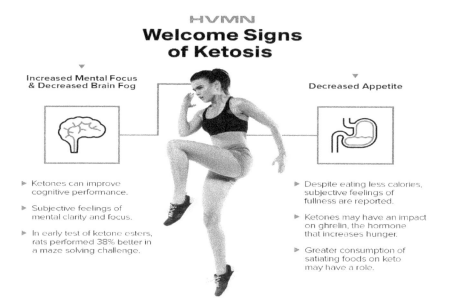

HVMN

Welcome Signs of Ketosis

Increased Mental Focus & Decreased Brain Fog

▶ Ketones can improve cognitive performance.

▶ Subjective feelings of mental clarity and focus.

▶ In early test of ketone esters, rats performed 38% better in a maze solving challenge.

Decreased Appetite

▶ Despite eating less calories, subjective feelings of fullness are reported.

▶ Ketones may have an impact on ghrelin, the hormone that increases hunger.

▶ Greater consumption of satiating foods on keto may have a role.

2.1   Bad breath

People also, after they hit complete ketosis, experience bad breath. It's a common side effect. Many individuals claim that their breath takes on a fruity scent on ketogenic diets and similar diets, such as the Atkins diet. Elevated levels of ketones cause it. Acetone, a ketone that leaves the body in the urine and respires, is the specific culprit (4Trusted Source). Although this breath can be less than optimal, it can be a good indicator of your social life diet. Many ketogenic dieters brush their teeth many times a day or use sugar-free gum to fix the issue. Check the carbohydrate mark if you use gum or other alternatives, such as sugar-free beverages. These will increase your blood sugar levels and decrease the level of ketones.

2.2 Loss of weight

Ketogenic diets are highly beneficial for weight loss and regular low-carb diets (5Trusted Source, 6Trusted Source). As hundreds of weight loss studies have shown, you will experience both short- and long-term weight loss (5Trusted Source, 7Trusted Source). During the first week, quick weight loss will occur. Although some individuals assume this is fat loss, carbs and water are mostly processed and used (8Trusted Source). It would help if you continued to lose body fat steadily as long as you adhere to the diet and stay in a calorie deficit after the initial rapid water weight decrease.

2.3 Increased blood ketones

A drop in blood sugar levels and an increase in ketones are among the ketogenic diet hallmarks. You will continue to burn fat and ketones as the primary fuel sources as you move deeper into a ketogenic diet. Measuring the blood ketone levels using a specialized meter is the most effective and precise way of measuring ketosis. You are calculating the amount of beta-hydroxybutyrate (BHB) in your blood tests your ketone levels. It is one of the major ketones in the bloodstream that is present. According to some experts on the ketogenic diet, nutritional ketosis is characterized as blood ketones ranging from 0.5–3.0 mmol/L.The most effective testing method is to calculate ketones in your blood, and it is used in most scientific studies. However, the main drawback is that a tiny pinprick is needed to draw blood from your finger.

What's more, it can be costly for test kits. Most individuals can only conduct one test per week or every other week for this purpose. Amazon has a strong range available if you'd like to try checking your ketones.

2.4 Increased breath or urine ketones

A breath analyzer is another means of testing blood ketone concentrations. It tracks acetone, one of the three major ketones found during ketosis in your blood (4Trusted Source, 10Trusted Source).

It gives you an idea of the ketone levels in your body when more acetone exits the body as you are in ketosis (11Trusted Source). It has been shown that the use of acetone breath analyzers is reasonably effective but less accurate than the system used to track blood. Measuring the presence of ketones in your urine regularly with special indicator strips is another good technique. These often calculate ketone's excretion through the urine and be a simple and cheap way to test the ketone levels every day. They're not considered very accurate, though.

2.5 Suppression of appetite

When adopting a ketogenic diet, several individuals experience reduced hunger. The explanations why this is happening are still being discussed. However, it has been proposed due to an increased intake of proteins and vegetables, along with improvements in the hunger hormones of your body. To suppress appetite, the ketones themselves can also affect the brain (13).

2.6 Increased energy and concentration

When you first begin a very low-carb diet, people sometimes experience brain fog, tiredness, and feeling sick. It is called the "low carb flu" or "keto flu." However, improved concentration and energy are also recorded by long-term ketogenic dieters. Your body has to adjust to burning more fat for food instead of carbs when you start a low-carb diet. A major part of the brain starts burning ketones instead of glucose as you get into ketosis. For this to start working properly, it can take a few days or weeks. Ketones are an incredibly effective source of fuel for your brain. They have also been studied to treat brain diseases and disorders such as concussion and memory loss in a medical setting (14Trusted Source, 15Trusted Source, 16Trusted Source). It is no surprise. Therefore, long-term ketogenic dieters also report increased comprehension and enhanced brain function (17Trusted Source, 18Trusted Source). It can also help regulate and maintain blood sugar levels by removing carbohydrates. It will increase attention more and boost brain activity.

2.7 Exhaustion in the short term

For novice dieters, the initial transition to a ketogenic diet may be one of the biggest problems. Weakness and fatigue can be among their well-known side effects. Before they get into complete ketosis and enjoy all of the long-term benefits, these also lead people to abandon the diet. These adverse reactions are normal. Your body is forced to switch to a new system after many decades of working on a carb-heavy fuel system. This transition doesn't happen instantly, as you would imagine. In general, it takes 7-30 days for you to be in complete ketosis. You may want to take electrolyte supplements to minimize fatigue during this turn.

Owing to the rapid reduction in your body's water content and the removal of refined foods, which may have added salt, electrolytes are also lost. Try having 1,000 mg of potassium and 300 mg of magnesium a day by adding these supplements.

2.8 Short-term output declines

Removing carbs can lead to general tiredness at first, as discussed above. It requires an initial reduction in exercise performance. It is mainly caused by the reduction in your muscles' glycogen reserves, which provide all types of high-intensity exercise with the key and most effective fuel source. Many ketogenic dieters claim that their performance returns to normal after several weeks. A ketogenic diet may also be effective in some forms of ultra-endurance sports and activities. Besides, there are more advantages, namely an improved capacity to burn more fat during exercise. One famous study showed that when they exercised, athletes who converted to a ketogenic diet burned as much as 230 percent more fat than athletes who did not practice this diet (19Trusted Source).

Although it is unlikely that a ketogenic diet can improve professional athletes' efficiency, it should be enough for general exercise and leisure sports once you become fat-adapted.

2.9 Digestive Questions

Generally, a ketogenic diet requires a significant shift in the types of foods that you consume. At the onset, digestive problems such as constipation and diarrhea are typical side effects. After the adjustment time, some of these problems should subside, but it may be important to be aware of various foods that may cause digestive problems. Also, make sure that you consume plenty of good low-carb veggies low in carbohydrates but still provide a ton of fiber.

Most notably, don't make the mistake of eating a diet deficient in variety. Doing that can increase your risk of nutrient deficiencies and digestive problems.

2.10 Sleeplessness

Sleep, particularly when they first change their diet, is one major problem for many ketogenic dieters. When they first will their carbohydrates significantly, many individuals experience insomnia or wake up at night. In a couple of weeks, however, this typically changes. Several long-term ketogenic dieters say that after transitioning to the diet, they sleep better than before.

2.11 Ketosis Meet Tips

There are a variety of ways you can securely and efficiently get into dietary ketosis.

- **Reduce to less than 20 grams of daily net carb intake:**

While you do not need to be this stringent, eating less than 20 grams of net carbs per day ensures that you can reach nutritional ketosis.

What does it look like with 20 grams of carb? To find out or try out our keto recipes and meal plans that limit carbs to less than 20 grams per day, use our visual guide. Try intermittent fasting: Going without eating for 16-18 hours can help you get into ketosis more quickly. It is simple to do by simply missing breakfast or dinner, which can feel very normal on an appetite-suppressing keto diet.

- **Do not fear fat:**

An essential and delicious part of ketogenic eating is eating plenty of fat!

Make sure that each meal contains a source of natural fat.

- **Cook with coconut oil:**

Coconut oil contains medium-chain fatty acids and natural fat that stay stable at high heat, improving ketone production and having other advantages. If possible, exercise will not have enough resources to participate in intense physical activity during the transition into ketosis. Just going for a brisk walk, though, can help you get into ketosis more easily.

Chapter 3: Regulations on Keto Diets

The diet requires high amounts of fat, a moderate amount of protein, and a very limited amount of carbs to be consumed. It's usually broken down to 75, 20, and 5%, respectively, of your daily calories. Compare that with the traditional American diet, generally 50 to 65 percent carbohydrates, and it is fair to assume that this is a very different way of eating. The ketogenic diet is a diet that pushes the body to ketosis, a state in which the body uses fat as a primary source of fuel (instead of carbohydrates). Your body will reach a state of ketosis in one to three days if you eat the foods that will get you there, she adds. Much of the calories you eat are from fat, with a little protein and very little carbohydrates throughout the diet. If you eat a very low-calorie diet, ketosis often occurs; think doctor-supervised,

FACTORS THAT AFFECT WEIGHT LOSS ON KETO

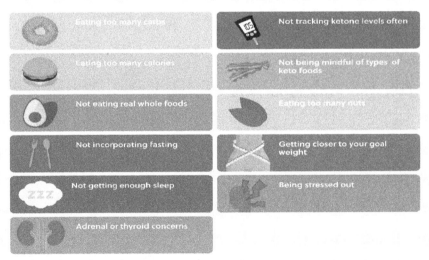

Eating too many carbs

Not tracking ketone levels often

Eating too many calories

Not being mindful of types of keto foods

Not eating real whole foods

Eating too many nuts

Not incorporating fasting

Getting closer to your goal weight

Not getting enough sleep

Being stressed out

Adrenal or thyroid concerns

PERFECT KETO

medically prescribed diets of 600 to 800 total calories per day.

3.1 Keto Guide to Food

Wondering what, and what doesn't, fit into a keto diet? "Knowing what foods you're going to eat before you start and how to incorporate more fats into your diet is so important,"

3.2 Seafood & Protein

Components:

- Mushrooms
- Garlic
- Green cabbage
- Green onions
- White onion
- Red bell pepper, red pepper
- Spinach
- Leaf or romaine lettuce
- Cherry tomatoes
- Avocado
- Lime

The Proteins

Components

- Boneless, Skinless Breasts Of Chicken
- Ground Beef
- Sausage For Breakfast
- Bacon

Eggs and milk

Components

- Cream cheese
- Eggs
- Single, whole-milk yogurt
- Blue cheese
- Salted butter

Staples from the pantry

Components

- Broth of chicken
- Cream of coconut
- Flour of almonds
- Soy sauce
- Extract vanilla
- Powder of cocoa
- Extract of monk fruit
- Almond butter
- Oils and spices
- Powder of garlic
- Salt
- Pepper
- Ground ginger
- Cinnamon
- Coconut oil

- Sesame oil

- Sesame seeds

- Oil for avocado

Seafood kinds of stuff

- Fish and other seafood prove to be incredibly good and nutritious.

- They are especially high in fatty acids such as B12, iodine, and omega-3, all nutrients that many people do not get enough of.

- Almost all types of fish and seafood contain almost no carbohydrates, just like beef.

The Salmon (Zero)

Salmon is, for a good reason, one of the most common fish types among health-conscious individuals.

It's a fatty fish, meaning that it contains significant amounts of heart-healthy fats, omega-3 fatty acids in this case.

Vitamin B12, iodine, and a decent amount of vitamin D3 are loaded with salmon as well.

Carbs: null

Trout style (Zero)

Like salmon, Trout is a type of fatty fish loaded with omega-3 fatty acids and other essential nutrients.

Carbs: null

Sardines (Zero)

Sardines are oily fish that, including their bones, are commonly eaten almost whole.

Sardines are among the world's most nutrient-dense foods and contain almost every single nutrient you need in your body.

Carbs: null

Shellfish (carbs of 4-5 percent)

It's a pity that shellfish barely make it onto people's daily menus since they are among the world's most healthy foods.

Currently, in their nutrient value, they rank similar to organ meats and are low in carbs.

Carbs: for every 100 grams of shellfish, 4-5 grams of carbs.

Certain Low-carb Shrimp and Fish

- Shrimps
- From Haddock
- Lobster-lobster
- The Herring
- The Tuna
- The Cod
- Catfish

3.3 Fat and Oil

- Oil from avocado
- Olive oil
- Coconut oil
- Butter
- Heavy cream

You have restricted your intake of these oils occasionally, which should be easy to do if you avoid processed foods, where they're sometimes contained.

- Sunflower oil

- Safflower oil

- Oil for corn

Never

- Margarine

- Artificial trans fats

3.4 Veggies and Fruits

- Avocado

- Leafy greens, including arugula and spinach

- Celery

- Asparagus

- Avocado

- Broccoli

- Cabbage

- Cauliflower

- Cucumber

- Green Beans

- Eggplant

- Kale

- Lettuce

- Olives

- Peppers (Especially Green

- Spinach
- Tomatoes
- Zucchini

These are decent options from time to time, but you'll need to count the carbs.

- Leeks
- Squash spaghetti
- Eggplant
- Potatoes
- Corn
- Raisins
- With broccoli (7 percent)
- Tomatoes and Tomatoes (4 percent)
- Onions (9 percent)
- Sprouts from Brussels (7 percent)
- Cauliflower Flower (5 percent)
- Kale (10 percent)
- Eggplants (6 percent)
- Cuckoo Cumber (4 percent)
- From Bell Peppers (6 percent)
- About asparagus (2 percent)
- The Green Beans (7 percent)
- Champignons (3 percent)
- Some Low-Carb Vegetables

- Celery

- Spinach

- Zucchini

- Swiss chard

- Cabbage

3.5 Seeds and Nuts

1. **Almonds:**2 grams of net carbs (6 grams total carbs)

2. **Brazil nuts:** net carbs of 1 gram (3 grams total carbs)

3. **Cashews:** 8 grams of total carbohydrates (9 grams total carbs)

4. **Macadamia nuts:** total carbs of 2 grams (4 grams total carbs)

5. **Pecans:**2 grams of net carbs (4 grams total carbs)

6. **Pistachios:** net carbs of 5 grams (8 grams total carbs)

7. **Walnuts:**2 grams of net carbs (4 grams total carbs)

8. **Chia seeds:** net carbs of 1 gram (12 grams total carbs)

9. **Pumpkin seeds:** net carbs of 3 grams (5 grams total carbs)

3.6 Dairy Products

- Blue cheese

- Brie

- Camembert

- Cheddar
- Chevre
- Colby Jack
- Cottage cheese
- Cream cheese
- Feta
- Goat's cheese
- Halloumi
- Havarti
- Limburger
- Manchego
- Mascarpone
- Mozzarella
- Muenster
- Parmesan
- Pepper Jack
- Provolone
- Romano
- String cheese
- Swiss
- Cheese from Cheddar
- Blue cheese
- Feta cheese
- Ice-cream

3.7 Sweetening agents

- Stevia

- Erythritol

- Xylitol

- Agave

- Honey

- Maple syrup

- White sugar and brown sugar

3.8 Sauces and Condiments

- Guacamole

- Sauce of lemon butter

- Mayonnaise (make sure no sugar is added)

- Raw garlic

- Tomato sauce (look for those with no added sugar) (look for those with no added sugar)

- Balsamic vinegar

- Barbecue sauce

- Ketchup

- Honey mustard

3.9 Drinks

- Water

- Milk of almonds

- Broth of bones

- Plain tea

- Black coffee (watch caffeine consumption)

- Carbonated water unsweetened (limit only if bubbles make you bloated)
- Soda diet
- Zero-calorie beverages
- Soda
- Fruit juice
- Lemonade

3.10 Spices and Herbs

Liberally, both herbs and spices work into a keto diet, but Mancinelli advises measuring the carbs if you use significant quantities.

- Salt (salt foods to taste)
- Pepper

Oregano, thyme, paprika, and cayenne

These are good options sometimes but do include some carbs.

- Ground ginger
- Powder of garlic
- Powder of Onion

No herbs and spices are off-limits; normally, they are okay to use in limited quantities to add flavor to foods.

3.11 Supplements

Consider needing to take

- Fiber

- Multivitamin

These are optional to help you generate ketones faster; Mancinelli says she has no advice to take or stop them.

- MCT oil

- Exogenous ketones

3.12 Cereals and bread

In many cultures, bread is a staple food. It comes in different types, such as loaves, bagels, rolls, and flatbreads, such as tortillas.

All of these are, however, high in carbs. It is true for types of whole grain as well as those made from processed flour. While carb counts vary depending on ingredients and portion sizes, the average numbers for common bread (1, 2, 3, 4) are as follows:

White bread (1 slice): 14 grams of carbohydrate, one fiber of which is

Whole-wheat bread (1 slice): 17 grams of carbohydrates, 2 of which are fiber-based.

10-inch flour tortilla: 36 grams of carbohydrates, 2 of which are fiber.

Bagel (3-inch): 29 grams of carbohydrates, 1 of which is fiber

Eating a sandwich, burrito, or bagel could bring you close to or over your daily limit, depending on your carb tolerance. Create your low-carb loaves at home if you do want to enjoy the bread. Most grains, including rice, wheat, and oats, are also high in carbs and, on a low-carb diet, need to be reduced or avoided.

3.13 Legumes and beans

Beans and legumes are nutritious crops. They can provide many health benefits, including decreased risk of inflammation and heart disease. While high in fiber, they contain a decent quantity of carbs as well. You may be able to use minor quantities on a low-carb diet, depending on personal tolerance. Here is the carb count for 1 cup (160-200 grams) of cooked beans and legumes.

1. **Lentils:** 40 grams of carbohydrates, of which 16 are fiber.

2. **Peas:** 25 grams of carbohydrates, nine of which are fiber.

3. **Black beans:** 41 grams of carbohydrates, of which 15 are fiber.

4. **Pinto beans:** 45 grams of carbohydrates, 15 of the fiber.

5. **Chickpeas:** 45 grams of carbohydrates, of which 12 are fiber.

6. **Kidney beans:** 40 grams of carbohydrates, 13 of the fiber.

3.14 List of Foods on the Keto Diet You Can't Eat:

- Grains
- Starchy vegetables and fruit with high sugar levels

- Yogurt sweetened

- Juices

- Any honey, syrup, or sugar

- Chips and crackers

- Baked products that include gluten-free baked goods

Chapter 4: Keto Diet Advantages & Risks

It is a complete understatement to say that the keto diet has become one of the most common diets in recent years. Case in point: There are over one million searches on Google every month for the keto diet. It's unique because people who want to lose weight have caught the fad diet's imagination, and there is no lack of recorded success stories to be found.

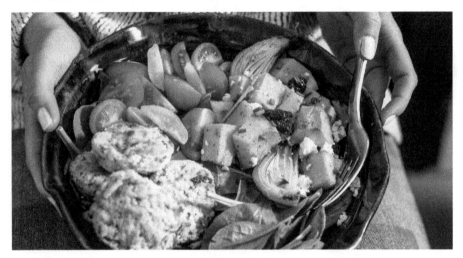

Reduce your hunger Low-carb diets

Controlling appetite

You would gain greater control of your appetite on a keto diet. For feelings of hunger to drop significantly, it is a very normal experience, and studies prove it.

Usually, this makes it easy to eat less and lose extra weight-just wait until you eat until you're hungry. It also makes it easier for intermittent fasting, which can boost attempts to cure type 2 diabetes and accelerate weight loss beyond the benefits of keto alone.

Plus, by not having to snack all the time, you could save time and money. On a keto diet (often skipping breakfast), many people feel the need to eat twice a day, and others only eat once a day, called OMAD. For issues such as sugar or food addiction, not having to battle hunger feelings may also theoretically help.

Finally, feeling fulfilled can be part of the solution. Food should stop being an enemy and become your friend or, whatever you want, simply fuel. The worst side effect of dieting appears to be hunger. It is one of the key reasons why many individuals feel miserable and give up eventually. A low-carb diet, however, results in an automatic decrease in appetite.

Studies have repeatedly shown that people eat much fewer calories when they cut carbs and consume more protein and fat.

Weight Loss Supports

In the first 3 to 6 months, a ketogenic diet might help you lose more weight than other diets. It may be because to turn fat into energy; requires more calories than it does to turn carbohydrates into energy. It's also likely that you are more comfortable with a high-fat, high-protein diet because you consume less, although that has not been confirmed yet. The ketogenic diet can encourage weight loss in many ways, including metabolism boosting and appetite reduction.

Ketogenic diets consist of foods that fill up a person and can decrease hormones that stimulate the appetite. For these reasons, it can decrease appetite and promote weight loss by adopting a keto diet.

Researchers found that individuals who adopted ketogenic diets lost 2 pounds (lbs.) more than those who followed low-fat diets over one year in a 2013 meta-analysis of 13 separate randomized controlled trials. Similarly, another study of 11 studies found that after six months, people who adopted a ketogenic diet lost 5 lbs. more than those who followed low-fat diets.

One of the easiest and most effective ways to lose weight is to cut carbohydrates. Studies indicate that people lose more weight quicker on low-carb diets than those on low-fat diets, even though the latter deliberately limits calories.

It is because low-carb diets work to rid the body of excess water, lower insulin levels and lead to rapid weight loss in the first week or two. In research contrasting low-carb and low-fat diets, individuals who reduce their carbohydrates often lose 2-3 times as much weight without being hungry/

Compared to a traditional weight loss diet, one study in obese adults showed a low-carb diet was particularly beneficial for up to six months. The difference in weight loss between diets was negligible after that. The two groups lost comparable amounts of weight in a year-long study of 609 overweight adults on low-fat or low-carb diets

Lowering the risk of such cancers

Researchers have studied the implications of the ketogenic diet to help avoid or even cure such cancers.

One study showed that in people with some diseases, a ketogenic diet could be a healthy and appropriate complementary medication to be used in addition to chemotherapy and radiation therapy. Cancer cells can cause more oxidative stress than normal cells, causing them to die.

More recent research from 2018 indicates that it may also reduce the risk of insulin complications because the ketogenic diet decreases blood sugar. Insulin is a blood sugar regulation hormone that may be linked to certain cancers.

While some research suggests that a ketogenic diet may benefit cancer treatment, there are limited studies in this field. Researchers need to perform further studies to fully appreciate the ketogenic diet's possible benefits in cancer prevention and care.

Blood sugar regulation and Type 2 reverse diabetes

Studies show that a ketogenic diet is excellent for type 2 diabetes management, sometimes even leading to a complete disease reversal.

It makes perfect sense, as keto reduces blood sugar levels, decreases the need for medication, and decreases the potentially negative effects of high insulin levels. Since a keto diet can reverse current type 2 diabetes and reverse pre-diabetes, it is likely to prevent it. Notice that the word "reversal" means that the condition improves and normalizes the glucose content in this sense.

In the best case, without the need for drugs, blood glucose returns to normal. Lifestyle modifications, however, only work when you do them. If a person returns to the lifestyle he or she had before type 2 diabetes appeared and advanced, it is likely to come back and develop again over time.

Improved markers for the well-being

Many studies indicate that low-carb diets boost several significant risk factors for heart disease, including the cholesterol profile, which contains cholesterol and triglycerides of high-density lipoprotein (HDL). The concentrations of total and low-density lipoprotein (LDL) cholesterol are typically modestly affected.

Improved blood sugar levels, insulin levels, and blood pressure are also common. These often improved markers are related to "metabolic syndrome," an insulin-resistant disease managed effectively by low-carb diets.

From your abdominal cavity comes a greater proportion of the fat loss. The fat in your body is not always the same. Fat is processed dictates how your health and disease risk are affected.

Subcutaneous fat, which is under the skin, and visceral fat, which accumulates in the abdominal cavity and is common for most overweight men, are the two main forms.

They appear to lodge visceral fat around the organs. Inflammation and insulin resistance are associated with excess visceral fat and can drive the metabolic dysfunction that is so prevalent in the West today (8).

To reduce your unhealthy fat, low-carb diets are very successful. It seems like a greater proportion of the fat people lose on low-carb diets comes from the abdominal cavity.

It will lead to a significantly decreased risk of heart disease and type 2 diabetes over time. Fat molecules that circulate in your bloodstream are triglycerides.

High fasting triglycerides, levels in the blood after an overnight fast, are well known to be a strong risk factor for heart disease. Carb consumption is one of the main drivers of high triglycerides in sedentary people, especially simple sugar fructose.

They appear to undergo a very drastic decrease in blood triglycerides when individuals cut carbohydrates

Low-fat diets, on the other hand, also cause triglycerides to increase.

Increased 'Good' HDL Cholesterol levels

The 'healthy' cholesterol is also called high-density lipoprotein (HDL). The higher the HDL levels compared to "bad" LDL, the lower the risk of heart disease

Eating fat is one of the easiest ways to boost "good" HDL levels, and low-carb diets contain many fats.

Therefore, it is unsurprising that HDL levels increase significantly on balanced, low-carb diets, whereas low-fat diets appear to increase only marginally or even decrease.

Reduced levels of Blood Sugar and Insulin

On a ketogenic diet, people with diabetes frequently report remarkable

decreases in blood sugar levels. For both type 1 and type 2 diabetes, this is true.

Indeed, hundreds of controlled studies show that a very low-carb diet helps regulate blood sugar and can have other health benefits).

17 out of 21 individuals on a ketogenic diet were able to discontinue or decrease the dosage of diabetes medication in a 16-week trial. The study participants have lost 19 pounds (8.7 kg) on average and decreased their waist circumference, triglycerides, and blood pressure.

People in the ketogenic community averaged a 0.6 percent decrease in HbA1c in a 3-month study comparing a ketogenic diet to a moderate-carb diet. An HbA1c below 5.7% was achieved by 12% of participants, which is considered natural.

For people with diabetes and insulin resistance, low-carb and ketogenic diets may also be especially effective, impacting millions worldwide

Studies show that reducing carbohydrates significantly reduces blood sugar and insulin levels.

Any people with diabetes who start a low-carb diet may need almost instantly to reduce their insulin dosage by 50 percent

Ninety-five percent had lowered or discontinued their glucose-lowering medicine within six months in one study in people with type 2 diabetes

Speak to your doctor before making adjustments to your carb intake if you take blood sugar medicine, as your dose can need to be changed to avoid hypoglycemia.

Can Reduce blood pressure

A major risk factor for many illnesses, including heart disease, stroke, and kidney failure, is elevated blood pressure or hypertension.

Low-carb diets are an efficient way to lower blood pressure, decreasing the risk of these diseases and allowing you to live longer.

Against metabolic syndrome, successful

Metabolic syndrome is a disorder that is closely linked to the risk of heart failure and diabetes.

Metabolic syndrome is a series of symptoms, including:

- Pelvic obesity
- High blood pressure
- High levels of fasting blood sugar

- Elevated triglycerides

"Low levels of HDL cholesterol "good.

A low-carb diet, however, is exceptionally effective in treating all five of these symptoms.

These conditions are nearly eliminated under such a diet.

Improved levels of 'Bad' LDL Cholesterol

It is much more likely that people with high "bad" LDL will have heart attacks.

The size of the particles is, however, important. A higher risk of heart disease is associated with smaller particles, while larger particles are associated with a lower risk.

Low-carb diets are shown to increase the size of "bad" LDL particles while reducing the total number of LDL particles in your bloodstream.

For several brain disorders, therapeutic

Your brain needs glucose, as only this type of sugar can be burned in some parts of it. That's why your liver produces glucose from protein if you don't eat any carbs.

Yet, a large part of your brain can also burn ketones formed during starvation or when carb intake is very low.

It is the mechanism behind the ketogenic diet, which has been used for decades to treat epilepsy in children who don't respond to drug treatment

In many cases, this diet can cure children of epilepsy. In one study, over half of the children on a ketogenic diet experienced a greater than 50 percent reduction in their number of seizures, while 16 percent became seizure-free

Very low-carb and ketogenic diets are now being studied for other brain conditions, including Alzheimer's and Parkinson's disease.

Owing to abnormal brain activity, epilepsy is a condition that causes seizures.

For certain individuals with epilepsy, anti-seizure drugs are successful. Others don't respond to the medications, however, or can't handle their side effects.

Epilepsy has by far the most data supporting it of all the disorders that may benefit from a ketogenic diet. Besides, there are several dozen studies on the subject.

Research indicates that in around 50 percent of epilepsy patients who adopt the classic ketogenic diet, seizures usually improve. It is often referred to as a ketogenic 4:1 diet because it contains four times as much fat as combined protein and carbs.

Beyond seizure prevention, the ketogenic diet can also help the brain.

For example, when researchers analyzed children with epilepsy's brain activity, 65 percent of those adopting a ketogenic diet found changes in different brain patterns, regardless of whether they had fewer seizures.

Polycystic Disease of Ovary (PCOS)

Polycystic ovary syndrome (PCOS) is a hormonal dysfunction-marked disorder that sometimes leads to irregular cycles and infertility.

Insulin resistance is one of its hallmarks, and many women with PCOS are obese and have a tough time losing weight. Women with PCOS often have an elevated chance of developing type 2 diabetes

Many that meet the metabolic syndrome criterion tend to have symptoms that impact their appearance. Effects can include increased hair on the face, acne, and other signs of masculinity associated with increased testosterone levels

It is possible to find a lot of anecdotal information online. However, just a few published studies affirm the advantages of low-carb and ketogenic PCOS diets

Weight loss averaged 12 percent in a six-month study of eleven women with PCOS following a ketogenic diet. Insulin fasting also decreased by 54 percent, and levels of reproductive hormones increased. Two infertility-suffering women became pregnant.

Adiposity

Many studies indicate that ketogenic, very low-carb diets are much more successful than calorie-restricted or low-fat diets for weight loss

What's more, they typically also make other wellness improvements.

Men who adopted a ketogenic diet lost twice as much weight in a 24-week study as men who consumed a low-fat diet

Furthermore, the ketogenic community's triglycerides dropped dramatically, and their HDL ("good") cholesterol increased. A smaller reduction in triglycerides and a decline in HDL cholesterol occurred in the low-fat population.

The capacity of ketogenic diets to minimize malnutrition is one reason they perform so well for weight loss.

A major study found that ketogenic diets, very low-carb, calorie-restricted, make people feel less hungry than usual calorie-restricted diets (66Trusted Source).

Even if people on a ketogenic diet can consume whatever they want, they usually end up consuming fewer calories due to ketosis's appetite-suppressing effects.

Those in the ketogenic community had substantially less appetite, took in fewer calories, and lost 31 percent more weight than the moderate-carb group in a study of obese men who consumed either a calorie-unrestricted ketogenic or moderate-carb diet.

Fatty Liver Nonalcoholic Disorder

The most common liver disease in the Western world is a nonalcoholic fatty liver disease (NAFLD).

Type 2 diabetes, metabolic syndrome, and obesity are closely related, and there is evidence that NAFLD also improves on a very low-carb, ketogenic diet.

In a small study, there were substantial reductions in weight, blood pressure, and liver enzymes in 14 obese men with metabolic syndrome and NAFLD following a ketogenic diet for 12 weeks

What's more, an incredible 93% of men had a reduction in liver fat, and 21% had a full NAFLD resolution.

Improving cardiac health

When a person follows a ketogenic diet, selecting healthy foods is important. Some evidence suggests that consuming healthier fats, such as avocados, can boost heart health by reducing cholesterol instead of less healthy fats, such as pork rinds.

A 2017 study of animal and human research on a keto diet found that some individuals experienced a substantial decrease in total cholesterol, low-density lipoprotein (LDL) or poor cholesterol and triglycerides levels, and a rise in high-density lipoprotein (HDL) or "good" cholesterol levels.

High cholesterol levels will increase the risk of cardiovascular disease. Therefore, a keto diet's decreasing effect on cholesterol may decrease the risk of heart complications for a person.

However, the analysis concluded that the beneficial effects of the diet on heart health depend on the diet's consistency. Thus, when following the keto diet, it is important to eat good, nutritionally balanced food.

Complications and threats

There can be a variety of health benefits to the ketogenic diet. However, a long-term stay on a ketogenic diet may have an adverse health effect, including an increased risk of the following health problems:

- Kidney Stones
- Excess protein in the blood
- Deficits of minerals and vitamins
- The deposition of fat in the liver

The keto diet can cause negative side effects that are known to many people as keto flu. These negative effects can include:

- Constipation
- Tiredness
- Low blood sugar levels
- Nausea
- Vomiting
- Headaches
- A poor exercise tolerance

At the beginning of the diet, these symptoms are particularly frequent as the body transitions to its new nutrition source.

The keto diet should be avoided by certain populations, including:

- Insulin-dependent people with diabetes
- Persons with eating disorders

- Those with pancreatitis or kidney failure
- During pregnancy and breastfeeding, females

A keto diet should also not be practiced by people who take a drug named sodium-glucose cotransporter 2 (SGLT2) inhibitor for type 2 diabetes. The risk of diabetic ketoacidosis, a dangerous disorder that increases acidity in the blood, is increased by this drug.

CHAPTER 5: Are you on the Keto Diet?

To lose weight, people use a ketogenic diet most often, but it can help manage certain medical conditions, such as epilepsy. People with heart disease, certain brain diseases, and even acne may also be helped, but more research in those areas needs to be done. To find out if it's safe for you to try a ketogenic diet, talk to your doctor first, especially if you have type 1 diabetes.

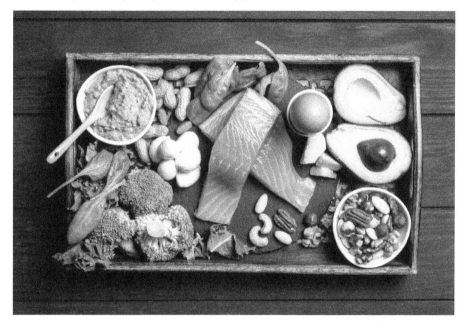

There are controversies and misconceptions concerning the keto diet, but it seems very healthy for most people.

Three classes, however, often need special consideration:

Do you take diabetes medicine, including insulin, for example?

Do you take high blood pressure medication?

Women's breastfeeding

However, under medical supervision, certain people should only follow a ketogenic diet, and others are best off avoiding it altogether.

Conditions that require medical monitoring and supervision during ketosis:

- Diabetes type 1
- Type 2 diabetes on treatment for insulin or oral diabetes
- High blood pressure on medications
- Liver, respiratory, or renal disorder
- History of surgery for gastric bypass
- Pregnancy
- Conditions for which it is important to prevent ketosis:
- Women breastfeeding

Individuals with unusual metabolic disorders commonly get diagnosed in infancy, such as defects in enzymes that interfere with the body's ability to produce and use ketones or digest fats properly.

Chapter 5: Keto diet with elevated blood pressure

So, you have high blood pressure, and you want to try a diet low in carbohydrates or keto? Oh, congratulations! It could be the most powerful thing for naturally reducing your blood pressure.

It can also completely normalize the blood pressure in some situations.

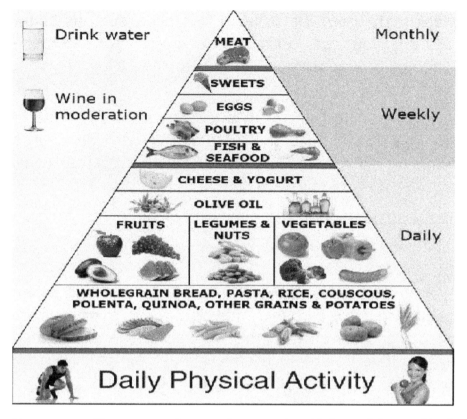

Drink water — Wine in moderation

Monthly — Weekly — Daily

MEAT
SWEETS
EGGS
POULTRY
FISH & SEAFOOD
CHEESE & YOGURT
OLIVE OIL
FRUITS | LEGUMES & NUTS | VEGETABLES
WHOLEGRAIN BREAD, PASTA, RICE, COUSCOUS, POLENTA, QUINOA, OTHER GRAINS & POTATOES

Daily Physical Activity

However, there are two minor potential problems that you will need to be aware of before you start.

1. Medication for blood-pressure

There is a chance of the diet working too well if you are on blood pressure medicine and start a low-carb diet! That may mean you have a low blood pressure history. It's true, yes. For your current drug dose, you can become too healthy.

With low-carb nutrition, this blood pressure-lowering effect may occur within days, but it can also take months or even a year to achieve its maximum effect.

You can immediately check your blood pressure if you experience signs of low blood pressure, such as feeling weak, exhausted, or dizzy. If it is poor, such as below 120/80, you can contact your doctor to determine whether it is acceptable for you to reduce or quit your medication.

It is something that most physicians should be able to do. But if you need to find a doctor with good drug handling skills on a low-carb diet, check out our chart and directory of low-carb doctors.

We also have a comprehensive blood pressure drug guide.

2. Bouillon and salt

We often suggest having extra fluid and salt when beginning a low-carb diet, maybe in the form of bouillon, particularly during the first two weeks. The explanation is to mitigate early side effects that may otherwise be problematic if low carb begins, e.g., headache.

This bouillon can only be taken if the blood pressure is well controlled, as it can slightly raise blood pressure for others.

If despite medicine, your blood pressure is high, you should not take extra salt or bouillon. Doing so could increase even higher blood pressure, and it is not prudent to risk that.

The good news is that when your body moves from using glucose to using fat as its primary fuel, any side effects will usually pass within days to a few weeks.

Keto Diabetic Diet

So, you have diabetes, and you want to try low-carb or keto foods? Pretty good for you! There is the ability to cure type 2 diabetes by making these lifestyle improvements. Or, if you have type 1 diabetes, doing so might increase your blood sugar regulation dramatically.

1.You need to know what you are doing, though, and you need to communicate with your healthcare team frequently. You will probably have to reduce your insulin doses and some other diabetes medications once you start eating low carb, frequently by quite a lot.

2.The need for medication to lower it decreases by avoiding the carbohydrates that raise your blood sugar level. Taking the same oral insulin or insulin-stimulating medication dose as you did before taking a low-carb diet could result in low blood sugar, which can potentially become hazardous.

When beginning this diet, you need to monitor your blood sugar regularly and change your medicine accordingly. It can always be done with the aid of a doctor or other medical professional with diabetes experience.

If you have diabetes and are treated by diet alone, the risk of low blood sugar with low carb levels is extremely low. You will instantly get started.

You would need to lower the doses as a general rule when beginning a strict low-carb diet.

3.Act on finding the best initial reduction with your doctor. Many notice that the decrease will need to be between 30 and 50%.

4.Consider reducing both doses by the same proportion if you take insulin once or twice daily. Your meal doses should be decreased first if you are on a basal-bolus regimen (taking fast-acting insulin before meals and long-acting insulin once or twice daily).

You will likely be able to avoid mealtime insulin entirely if you stay low carb. If your blood sugar levels stay steady, you may then begin decreasing your long-acting insulin.

5.Many individuals on a low-carb diet are entirely capable of going off insulin.

6.Sadly, there is no way to know how much insulin is needed in advance. Based on your blood sugar readings, you'll have to monitor your blood sugar regularly and lower insulin doses. With the help of a competent doctor or healthcare staff, this should be done.

Notice that many believe it's easier to err on the low side of insulin doses, as a general rule. You will later take more insulin to help get it down if your blood sugar goes a little high. That's good.

7.That's much riskier if you take too much insulin instead and end up with low sugar.

To lift your sugar to a healthy amount, you would also have to rapidly consume or drink glucose or some form of rapid-acting carbohydrate, which possibly decreases the impact of a low-carb diet.

For type 1 diabetes, insulin

Most of the insulin guidance above also applies to persons with type 1 diabetes. To help people with type 1 diabetes get healthy blood sugars, a low-carb, high-fat diet can be awesome.

8.It also results in far fewer and milder highs or hypos, as long as insulin doses are sufficiently decreased.

9.However, eating low-carb with type 1 diabetes requires even more attention to blood sugar levels and insulin change and an even closer working relationship between you and your health care team. To help you discuss future changes with your doctor, this section will review general guidelines.

Many people with type 1 diabetes use their mealtime insulin with an insulin-to-carbohydrate ratio (ICR). In this scenario, you can continue to give the same ratio of insulin to the carbohydrates you eat with a low-carb diet. However, you can automatically inject less total insulin when you eat fewer carbohydrates.

Due to protein increasing insulin requirements, a higher ICR may be needed in certain cases.

10.A lower ICR may be required in other cases. On a low-carb diet, certain individuals will lose weight and become more insulin sensitive. If this happens, the insulin to carbohydrate ratio, and likely even the basal insulin doses, may need to be decreased.

People who use relatively fixed mealtime insulin doses or those who use insulin twice daily should use the same type 2 diabetes strategy. Of course, the difference is that people with type 1 diabetes and a very low carbohydrate diet will still require some insulin.

It is important to be aware that ketosis can result from a diet with less than 50 grams of carbs per day. It is a normal physiological state resulting from the energy-burning of fat by the body.

Relatively high but still physiological (in other words, safe) ketone levels (e.g., between 0.5 and 3.0 mmol/L, but sometimes as high as 4 or 5 mmol/L) can result from a very strict low-carb diet. It should not be confused with ketoacidosis, a dangerous complication of type 1 diabetes when insufficient insulin is present.

11.The normal response to using fat for energy is ketosis. It's fine for healthy individuals, but this means you need to be sure that you can distinguish ketosis from the much more dangerous ketoacidosis in type 1 diabetes. High blood sugar levels and dehydration, as well as high ketones, are associated with the latter.

Therefore, we recommend that a person with type 1 diabetes starts with a more liberal low-carb diet when starting low-carb diet, with at least 50 grams of carbs a day.

12.If you wish, while working closely with your healthcare team and carefully monitoring your ketone levels, you can then begin to decrease your carb intake to 30-40 grams of carbs per day.

We do not recommend starting a low-carb ketogenic diet (less than 20 grams a day) unless you know how to deal with this risk and work closely with a very experienced healthcare professional. If you feel even slightly ill, practice intermittent fasting, or have been exercising, you also have to be able to test your ketones frequently and use additional care.

13.It is also important to remember that while individuals with type 2 diabetes can often reverse their illness sufficiently to stop taking insulin injections completely, someone with type 1 diabetes will always have to replace the insulin they lack.

Chapter 6: Recipes

6.1 Coffee from Keto

INGREDIENTS

- 1 cup Hot black coffee, freshly brewed
- 1 tablespoon butter or ghee fed with grass
- 1 1/2 teaspoons Oil for MCT

INSTRUCTIONS

In a blender, position 1 cup of brewed coffee, one tablespoon of butter or ghee, and 1 1/2 teaspoons of MCT oil and blend at high speed for about 30 seconds until emulsified, frothy, and lightened in color.

KETO DIET
FOOD PYRAMID

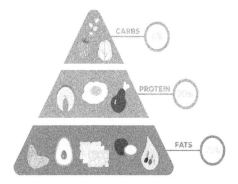

6.2 Keto Chicken Salad

INGREDIENTS

- 1.5 lb breast of chicken

- 3 celery ribs, diced

- 1/2 cup of mayo

- 2 tsp of brown mustard

- 1/2 Tsp Himalayan pink salt
- 2 tbsp of fresh dill, chopped

- 1/4 cup of pecans chopped

INSTRUCTIONS

1. Preheat the oven to 450 ° F and line the parchment paper baking sheet.

2. Bake the chicken breast until cooked, around 15 minutes or so.

3. Take the chicken out of the oven and let it cool. Break the chicken into bite-sized pieces after it has cooled completely.

4. Put the chicken, celery, mayo, brown mustard, and salt in a big bowl. Toss once you have thoroughly coated the chicken and the ingredients are well mixed.

5. Cover the bowl with a lid or plastic wrap and refrigerate for around 1-2 hours until chilled.

6. Add fresh dill and chopped pecans when ready to eat, and toss gently. Serve refrigerated and enjoy.

6.3 Crisps with Keto Cheese

INGREDIENTS

- Cheddar grass-fed cheese

- 1 Jalapeno medium-sized

- 2 bacon slices

INSTRUCTIONS

1. Preheat the oven to 425 ° F and line a baking sheet with a silicone baking mat or parchment paper.

2. Apply to the prepared baking sheet, also heaped tablespoons of cheese. Place one jalapeno slice in the middle of the mound. We are using crumbled bacon to sprinkle.

3. Bake for 7-10 minutes on warm until the cheese melts and the edges are browned.

4. Remove from the oven and allow to cool until crisp fully.

6.4 Stew of Keto Beef

INGREDIENTS

- 2 lb. Roasted beef chuck, sliced into 1-inch sections
- Salt of Kosher
- Black pepper freshly ground.
- For 2 tbsp. Olive Oil Extra-Virgin
- 8 of an oz. Baby mushrooms Bella, sliced
- 1 Tiny onion, chopped
- 1 medium carrot, peeled and sliced into circles.
- 2 Celery Stalks, Cut
- 3 Garlic cloves, minced

- For 1 tbsp. Paste of tomatoes
- 6 c. Low-sodium broth for beef
- For 1 tsp. New leaves of thyme
- For 1 tsp. Rosemary Newly Chopped

INSTRUCTIONS

1. With paper towels, pat beef dry and salt and pepper season well. Heat oil in a large pot over medium heat. Working in lots, add beef and sear on all sides until golden, around 3 minutes per side. Remove from the pot and repeat with remaining beef, adding more oil as needed.

2. Add mushrooms to the same pot and cook for 5 minutes until golden and crispy. Add onion, carrots, and celery and cook for 5 minutes until tender. Add garlic and cook 1 minute more, until fragrant. Add tomato paste and stir to coat vegetables.

3. To the pot, add broth, thyme, rosemary, and beef and season with salt and pepper. Bring to a boil and reduce heat to a simmer. Simmer 50 minutes to an hour until beef is tender.

6.5 Keto Cabbage Stuffed

INGREDIENTS

THE SAUCE FOR:

- 1 Tomato can be diced (14-oz.)
- For 1 tbsp. Vinegar Apple Cider
- 1/2 tsp. Flakes of red pepper
- For 1 tsp. Powdered onion
- For 1 tsp. Powdered garlic
- For 1 tsp. Oregano dried
- Salt of Kosher

- Black pepper freshly ground.
- 1/4 of a c. Olive Oil Extra-Virgin
- For the rolls of cabbage:
- 12 Leaves for cabbage
- With 1 lb. Ground-based beef
- From 3/4 lb. Pork Field
- 1 of a c. Riced Cauliflower Flowers
- 3 Thinly sliced green onions
- 1/4 of a c. Parsley chopped, plus more for serving.
- Black pepper freshly ground.

INSTRUCTIONS

FOR THE SAUCE :

1. preheat oven to 375 ° C. In a blender, purée tomatoes, apple cider vinegar, red pepper flakes, onion powder, garlic powder, and oregano; salt and pepper seasoning.

2. Heat oil over medium heat in a large deep skillet (or large pot). Add pureed tomato sauce, bring to a boil, lower to medium-low, and simmer for 20 minutes, until thickened slightly.

For the rolls of cabbage:

1. Blanch cabbage leaves until tender and flexible, approximately 1 minute, in a large pot of boiling water. Set aside.

2. Make the filling: mix 1/2 c. tomato sauce, ground beef, cauliflower rice, scallions, and parsley in a large bowl. Season with salt and pepper.

3. On the bottom of a large baking dish, spread a thin layer of sauce. Cut out the hard triangular rib from each cabbage leaf using a paring knife. Put about 1/3 cup filling into one end of each leaf, then roll up, tucking in

the sides as you roll. Place seam rolls side-down in baking dish on top of sauce. Spoon remaining sauce on top of cabbage rolls. Bake until the meat is 45 minutes to 55 minutes

4. Garnish before serving with more parsley.

6.6 Keto Casserole for Breakfast

INGREDIENTS

- 6 slices of bacon
- 12 large eggs
- 4 oz. of sour cream
- 4 oz. Heavy whipping cream
- To taste salt & pepper
- Cooking spray for avocado oil
- 10 oz. cheddar cheese shredded
- 1/3 cup of green onions, chopped (optional garnish)

INSTRUCTIONS

1. Preheat a 350 ° F oven.

2. Cook bacon on a stovetop. Crumble into bite-sized bits until cooked and cooled.

3. Smash eggs in a medium-sized bowl. Add sour cream, heavy whipping cream, salt, and pepper and mix until well-combined with a hand mixer or in a blender.

4. Spray avocado oil cooking spray with a 9-13 plate. Arrange a single layer of cheddar cheese to the pan.

5. Pour egg mixture on top of the cheese, then top with crumbled bacon.

6. Bake for 35 minutes, checking after 30 minutes. Once the casserole edges are golden brown, remove them from the oven.

7. Before cutting and serving, leave to cool. Garnish with green onions.

6.7 Greek Chicken Garlicky

INGREDIENTS

- 3 tbsp. Extra virgin olive oil, split-up
- Juice with one lemon
- 3Garlic cloves, minced
- 1 tsp. Oregano dried with 1 lb. Thighs of Chicken
- Kosher salt, Black pepper freshly ground.
- 1/2 lb Asparagus removed ends.
- 1Sliced into half-moons of zucchini
- 1Sliced lemon

INSTRUCTIONS

1. Mix 2 tablespoons of olive oil, lemon juice, garlic, and oregano in a large bowl. Whisk until mixed, then add chicken thighs and toss to coat. Cover the bowl with plastic wrap and allow to marinate for at least 15 minutes and up to 2 hours in the refrigerator.

2. Preheat the oven to 425 ° when the chicken is ready to cook. Heat the remaining tablespoon of olive oil in a large oven-proof skillet over medium-high heat. Season the marinated chicken with salt and pepper on both sides, then add the chicken skin-side down and pour in the remaining marinade.

3. Sear for about 10 minutes until the skin becomes golden and crispy. Rotate the chicken and add the asparagus, zucchini, and lemons to the skillet.

4. Move the pan to the oven and cook for about 15 minutes until the chicken is cooked and the vegetables are tender.

6.8 Muffins with Keto Egg

INGREDIENTS

Olive oil or cooking spray

- 1/2 cups Sweet Potato Shredded (from about one medium potato)
- 1 cup Shredded cheddar strong cheese (about 4 ounces)
- 6 Fried strips of sugar-free, crumbled bacon
- 10 Large-sized eggs
- 1/4 of a cup the Half
- 1 teaspoon Kosher salt,
- 1/4 of a teaspoon Black pepper, freshly roasted

INSTRUCTIONS

1. In the middle of the oven, arrange a rack and heat to 400 ° F. Coat a 12-well regular muffin tin with cooking spray or olive oil generously. Divide the sweet potato, cheese, and bacon shredded equally between the muffin wells.

2. In a wide bowl, put the eggs, half-and-half, salt, and pepper and whisk until the eggs are fully incorporated. Pour into the muffin wells, filling every 1/2 to 3/4.

3. Bake for 12 to 14 minutes until the muffins are set and lightly browned around the edges. Position the pan on a wire rack and allow 2 to 3 minutes to cool. Run a butter knife around each cup to loosen the muffins before removing them from the pan. Before cooling or freezing, serve warm or cool completely on a wire rack.

6.9 Bread Keto Loaf

INGREDIENTS

- Two cups Fine ground almond flour, such as brands from Bob's Red Mill or King Arthur

- 1 teaspoon Powder for baking

- 1/2 teaspoon of tea Gum xanthan

- 1/2 teaspoon of tea

- Kosher salt
- 7 large eggs at room temperature,
- Eight tablespoons (1 stick) melted and cooled unsalted butter
- Two tablespoons Melted and cooled refined coconut oil

INSTRUCTIONS

1. In the center of the oven, arrange a rack and heat it to 350°F. Line the bottom and sides of a parchment paper 9x5-inch metal loaf pan, letting the excess hang over the long sides to form a sling. Only set aside.

2. In a medium cup, whisk together the almond flour, baking powder, xanthan gum, and salt. Only set aside.

3. Place the eggs in a bowl fitted with the whisk attachment of a stand mixer. Beat until light and frothy, at the medium-high level. Lower the speed to medium, add the melted butter and coconut oil slowly, and beat until well mixed. Reduce the speed to medium, add the mixture of almond flour slowly, and beat until mixed. Increase the speed to medium and beat for around 1 minute before the mixture thickens.

4. Pour the prepared pan into it and smooth out the end. Bake for 45 to 55 minutes until a knife inserted in the middle comes out clean. Let it cool for about 10 minutes in the pan. Remove the loaf from the pan, grab the

parchment paper, and transfer it to a wire rack. Until slicing, cool absolutely.

6.10 Keto balls of meat

INGREDIENTS

- 1 lb. Ground-based beef
- 1 big egg
- 1/2 cup of grated parmesan
- 1/2 cup of mozzarella shredded
- 1 tbsp of minced garlic
- 1 T.L. of black pepper
- 1/2 tsp of salt
- 1 scoop of Whey Protein Great Keto Unflavored (optional)

INSTRUCTIONS

1. Preheat the oven to 400°C—line a parchment paper baking sheet.

2. Combine all the ingredients in a mixing bowl with your hands and knead until well incorporated.

3. Shape the mixture into meatballs of the same size and put them on the prepared baking sheet.

4. For 18-20 minutes, bake.

5. Enable slightly to cool and serve warm.

6.11 Mac & Cheese Keto

INGREDIENTS

- Butter, for dish baking
- 2 Cauliflower Medium Heads, cut into florets.
- For 2 tbsp. Olive Oil Extra-Virgin
- Salt of Kosher
- 1 of a c. Heavy milk to heavy cream

- Oh. 6 oz. Cheese cream, cut into cubes.
- Oh. 4 c. Cheddar Shredded
- Oh. 2 c. Mozzarella Sliced
- For 1 tbsp. Hot Sauce Hot Sauce (optional)
- Black pepper freshly ground.
- For the Topper
- 4 of an oz. Rinds of pork, crushed
- 1/4 of a c. Parmesan, freshly grated
- For 1 tbsp. Olive Oil Extra-Virgin
- For 2 tbsp. For garnish, finely chopped parsley

INSTRUCTIONS

1. Preheat the oven to 375 ° and cook a 9"-x-13" baking dish with butter. Toss the cauliflower with two tablespoons of oil in a wide bowl and season with salt. On two large baking sheets, spread the cauliflower and roast until tender and softly golden for about 40 minutes.

2. Meanwhile, over medium heat, heat the cream in a large pot. Bring to a boil, then reduce heat to medium, and when melted, whisk in the cheeses. When using, remove from the oven, add hot sauce, and season with salt and pepper; fold in the roasted cauliflower. If needed, taste and season more.

3. Move the blend to the ready-made baking dish. Stir to mix the pork rinds, parmesan, and oil in a medium dish. Sprinkle the mixture over the cauliflower and cheese in an even layer.

4. Bake for 15 minutes, until golden. Switch the oven to broil to toast more, around 2 minutes if needed.

5. Until serving, garnish it with parsley.

6.12 Chicken Sunny Chicken

INGREDIENTS

- For 1 tbsp. Olive Oil Extra-Virgin
- 6 The bone-in, skin-on thighs of chicken (about 2 pounds)
- Salt of Kosher
- Black pepper freshly ground.
- 2 Garlic cloves, minced
- For 1 tbsp. New leaves of thyme
- For 1 tsp. Crushed flakes of red pepper
- 3/4 of c. Low-sodium broth for chicken
- 1/2 of a c. Heavy milk to heavy cream
- 1/2 of a c. Sun-dried tomatoes chopped
- 1/4 of a c. Parmesan, freshly grated
- Basil, freshly torn, for serving.

INSTRUCTIONS

1. Preheat the oven to 375 degrees. Heat the oil in a big oven-safe skillet over medium-high heat. With salt and pepper, season chicken generously and sear, skin-side down, until golden, 4 to 5 minutes on each side. Place the chicken on a plate and pour half of the fat out of the skillet.

2. Bring the skillet back to medium heat and apply the flakes of garlic, thyme, and red pepper. Cook for 1 minute until fragrant, then stir in the broth, heavy cream, sun-dried tomatoes, and Parmesan cheese and add more salt to taste. Bring the chicken to a boil, then return it to the skillet, skin-side-up.

3. Move the skillet to the oven and bake for 17 to 20 minutes until the chicken is cooked (and the juices run clear when the chicken is pierced with a knife).

4. Garnish and serve with basil.

6.13 Provençale keto chicken

INGREDIENTS

- 2 lbs. of chicken legs
- 8 oz. Tomatoes (11/4 cups)
- 21/2 oz. (1/2 cup) black, pitted olives
- 1/4 cup of olive oil
- 5 cloves of garlic, cut
- 1 tbsp oregano dried
- Salt and pepper

To represent

- 7 oz. Lettuce (51/2 cups)

- 1 cup of mayonnaise

- 1/4 lemon, zest

- 1 tsp of powder paprika

- Salt and pepper

INSTRUCTIONS

1. Preheat the furnace to 200 °C (400 °F). Place your chicken skin in an oven-proof baking dish on the side. On top of and around the beef, add garlic, olives, and tomatoes.

2. Drizzle the olive oil with a generous amount. Season with salt and pepper and sprinkle with oregano.

3. Put in the oven until the chicken is completely cooked through and roast. Depending on the size of the pieces, it should take about 45-60 minutes. If you feel uncertain, use a meat thermometer to check the internal temperature. When the temperature exceeds 180 ° F (75 ° C), the chicken is cooked.

4. Serve with lemon zest and paprika or mild chili and some salt and pepper flavored salad and mayo.

6.14 Cups for Pizza
INGREDIENTS

- 12 slices of deli ham
- 1 lb. Italian sausage in bulk
- 12 tbsp pizza sauce sugar-free
- 3 cups of mozzarella cheese grated
- 24 slices of pepperoni
- 1 cup of bacon cooked and crumbled

INSTRUCTIONS

1. Preheat the furnace to 375 F. Italian brown sausage in a frying pan, draining the extra fat.

2. Line the 12-cup muffin tray with slices of ham. Between each cup, divide the sausage, pizza sauce, mozzarella cheese, pepperoni slices, and bacon crumbles in that order.

3. Bake for 10 minutes at 375. Broil until the cheese bubbles and browns, and the edges of the meat toppings look crispy for 1 minute.

4. Remove the pizza cups from the muffin tin and place them on a paper towel to avoid wetting the bottoms. Sip instantly or refrigerate and reheat in the microwave or toaster oven.

6.15 Chicken's Cheesy Bacon Ranch

INGREDIENTS

- 4 Thick-cut bacon slices
- 4 Chicken breasts with boneless skinless skin (about 1 3/4 lbs.)
- Salt of Kosher
- Black pepper freshly ground.
- Seasoning for the ranch
- 1 1/2 of a c. Mozzarella Sliced
- Chopped chives for decoration

INSTRUCTIONS

1. Cook bacon, flipping once, in a large skillet over medium heat, until crispy, around 8 minutes. Transfer to a plate-lined paper towel. Drain all but two tablespoons of the skillet's bacon fat.

2. Season the chicken with pepper and salt. Return the skillet to medium-high heat, add the chicken and cook for around 6 minutes per side until golden and just cooked through.

3. Reduce heat to medium and top with mozzarella and sprinkle chicken with ranch seasoning. Cover the skillet and cook for about 5 minutes until the cheese is melted and bubbly.

4. Before serving, crumble and scatter the bacon and chives on top.

6.16 Spinach-Mozzarella Burgers Stuffed
INGREDIENTS

- Make four patties, enough for four people,
- Ground chuck 11/2 lbs.
- One salt teaspoon
- 3/4 black pepper ground teaspoon
- 2 cups of fresh, firmly packed spinach
- 1/2 cup of mozzarella cheese shredded (about 4 oz)
- Two tablespoons of Parmesan cheese grated

INSTRUCTIONS

1.Combine the ground beef, salt, and pepper in a medium bowl.

2.Scoop around 1/3 cup of mixture and shape into eight patties about 1/2-inch thick with dampened hands. Could you place it in the fridge?

3.Place spinach over medium-high heat in a saucepan. Cover and cook until wilted for 2 minutes.

4.Let it drain and cool. Squeeze the spinach with your hands to remove as much liquid as possible.

5.Switch the spinach to a cutting board, chop it, and put it in a bowl.

6.Stir in the cheese and parmesan mozzarella.

7.Scoop about 1/4 cup of stuffing and mound four patties in the center,

8.Cover with the remaining four patties and, by pressing tightly together, seal the edges.

9.To round out the edges, cup each patty with your hands and press on the top to flatten slightly into a single thick patty.

10.Heat a grill or a grill pan to medium-high (lightly oil the grill grates if you are using an outdoor grill).

11.Grill the burgers on both sides for 5 to 6 minutes.

6.17 Garlic-butter roasted chicken legs and cherry tomatoes

INGREDIENTS

- 11/4 lbs. chicken legs
- 4 tablespoons olive oil
- 2 tbsp of seasoning in Italy
- Black pepper salt and ground
- 20 oz. With broccoli
- 20 oz. Tomatoes with Cherry Tomatoes Butter on Garlic
- 4 oz. Butter
- 2 cloves of garlic, pressed salt, and black ground pepper, to taste, serving
- 2 tbsp of fresh, chopped parsley (optional)

INSTRUCTIONS

1. Preheat the oven to around 200 °C (400 °F).

2. Toss the legs of the chicken with olive oil and season.

3. Together with the tomatoes, place the chicken legs, skin side up in a baking dish. Bake for 40-45 minutes or until the juices are clear and the chicken is 74 ° C (165 ° F).

4. Cut the broccoli into florets while the chicken is in the oven and cut the stem into slices (or use frozen). In a saucepan, boil in finely salted water for 5 minutes. To keep wet, drain the water and put on the lid.

5. Mix all the ingredients in a bowl of garlic butter. Only set aside.

6. Serve the broccoli, tomatoes, and garlic butter with the chicken.

6.18 Keto Salad with Eggs

INGREDIENTS

• 7 large whole eggs (hard-boiled, peeled, finely chopped)

• 1/2 cup of mayonnaise

• 1 T.L. of lemon juice

• 1 mustard teaspoon

1/4 of a cup of green onions (thinly sliced)

• 2 celery stalks (finely chopped)

• 1/2 teaspoon of salt

• 1/4 teaspoon of pepper

INSTRUCTIONS

1. To a medium-sized bowl, add all ingredients until thoroughly mixed.

2. Change the seasoning as you wish.

3. Refrigerate or instantly serve.

4. If needed, garnish it with extra green onions.

6.19 Keto Fried Chicken

INGREDIENTS

The Chickens

• 6Bone-in, skin-on breasts of chicken (about 4 lbs.)
• Salt of Kosher
• Black pepper freshly ground.
• 2 Large-sized eggs

- 1/2 of a c. Heavy milk to heavy cream
- 3/4 of c. Almond Flour
- 1 1/2 of a c. Finely crushed rinds of pork
- 1/2 of a c. Parmesan, freshly grated
- 1 tsp. Powdered garlic
- 1/2 tsp. Tweet Paprika
- 1/2 of a c. Mayonnaise
- 1 1/2Tsp.Hot Sauce

INSTRUCTIONS

1. Preheat the oven to 400 degrees and use parchment paper to line a large baking sheet. Pat the chicken dry with paper towels and salt and pepper to taste.

2. Whisk together the eggs and heavy cream in a shallow dish. Combine the almond flour, pork rinds, parmesan, garlic powder, and paprika in another shallow dish. With salt and pepper, season.

3. Dip the chicken into the egg mixture and then into the almond flour mixture one at a time, pressing to cover. Place the chicken on a ready-made baking sheet.

4. Bake for 45 minutes until the chicken is golden and the internal temperature reaches 165 °.

5. Meanwhile, make the dipping sauce: Blend the mayonnaise and hot sauce in a medium dish. Depending on the preferred amount of spiciness, add more hot sauce.

6. Serve warm chicken with sauce and dip.

6.20 Pesto Chicken Baked
INGREDIENTS

- Approximately 4 1.5 lb chicken breasts, cut in half widthwise to make eight parts.
- 3 tbsp of basil pesto
- Thinly sliced or shredded 8 oz mozzarella 1/2 tsp salt
- 1/4 tsp of black pepper

INSTRUCTIONS

1. Preheat the furnace to 350 F

2. Using cooking spray to spray the baking dish. Place the chicken in a single layer on the bottom and sprinkle it with salt and pepper. On the chicken, spread the pesto. On top, put the mozzarella.

3. Bake until the chicken is 160 degrees and the cheese is golden and bubbly, for 35-45 minutes. You can broil it at the end for a couple of minutes to brown the cheese if you like.

6.21 Chicken Stuffed Primavera

INGREDIENTS

- 4Skinless, boneless chicken breasts (approximately 1 1/2 pounds)
- 1 Zucchini, lengthwise halved and cut thinly into half-moons.
- 3 Halved and thinly sliced medium tomatoes into half-moons
- 2 Yellow bell peppers cut thinly.
- 1/2 Red onion, sliced thinly
- For 2 tbsp. Olive Oil Extra-Virgin
- For 1 tsp. Seasoning Italian
- Salt of Kosher
- Black pepper freshly ground.
- Mozzarella Sliced

- For garnish, finely chopped parsley

INSTRUCTIONS

1. Preheat the oven to 400 degrees. In each chicken breast, make slits, be careful not to cut through fully, and stuff them with zucchini, tomatoes, bell peppers, and red onion.

2. Drizzle with oil and season with salt, pepper, and Italian seasoning. We are using mozzarella to sprinkle.

3. Bake for 25 minutes until the chicken is completely cooked and no longer pink inside.

4. Until serving, garnish it with parsley.

6.22 Salad with Keto broccoli

INGREDIENTS

- 3 Broccoli heads, sliced into bite-size fragments
- 1/2 of a c. Cheddar Shredded
- 1:4 Red onion sliced thinly
- 1/4 of a c. Sliced almonds toasted
- 3 Slices of fried and crumbled bacon
- 2 tbsp. Chives that are newly chopped

For Dressing

- 2/3 of c. Mayonnaise
- 3 tbsp. Vinegar Apple Cider
- For 1 tbsp. Mustard
- kosher salt
- Black pepper freshly ground.

INSTRUCTIONS

1. Bring the 6 cups of salted water to a boil in a medium pot or saucepan. Prepare a big bowl of ice water while waiting for the water to boil.

2. Add the broccoli florets to the boiling water and cook for 1 to 2 minutes, until tender. With a slotted spoon, extract and put in the prepared ice water cup. Drain the florets in a colander when it is cold.

3. In a medium cup, whisk together the dressing ingredients—season with salt and pepper to taste.

4. In a big bowl, mix all the salad ingredients and pour over the dressing. Toss until the ingredients in the dressing are mixed and thoroughly coated. To eat, refrigerate until ready.

6.23 Rosemary Pork Chops with Garlic

INGREDIENTS

- 4 Pork chops loin
- Kosher salt
- Black pepper freshly ground.
- 1 tbsp. Rosemary freshly minced
- 2 Garlic cloves, minced
- 1/2 of a c. (1 stick) melted butter
- For 1 tbsp. Olive Oil Extra-Virgin

INSTRUCTIONS

1. Preheat the oven to 375 degrees F. With salt and pepper, season the pork chops generously.

2. Mix the butter, rosemary, and garlic in a small cup. Only set aside.

3. Heat the olive oil in an oven-safe skillet over medium-high heat and add the pork chops. Sear until golden, 4 minutes, flip and cook for an additional four minutes. Pork chops are generously coated with garlic butter.

4. Place the skillet in the oven and cook for 10-12 minutes, until cooked (145 ° for medium). Add more garlic butter to serve.

6.24 High-Protein Cottage Cheese Omelet

INGREDIENTS

- 2 Large-sized eggs
- 1 tablespoon whole or 2 percent milk
- 1/8 teaspoon Kosher salt
- Pinch freshly ground black pepper
- 1/2 tablespoon unsalted butter
- 1 cup baby spinach (about 1 ounce) (about 1 ounce)
- 3 tablespoonsCabin Cheese

INSTRUCTIONS

1. In a medium bowl, put the eggs, milk, salt, and pepper and whisk until the whites and yolks are thoroughly mixed, and the eggs are a little frothy.

2. Melt the butter over medium-low heat in an 8-inch nonstick frying pan. Tilt the pan so the butter coats the bottom evenly. Add the spinach and cook for about 30 seconds until it is wilted. Pour the eggs in and turn the pan immediately so that the eggs cover the entire bottom.

3. To gently drag and force the cooked eggs from the edges toward the middle of the pan, use a rubber or silicone spatula, allowing room for the uncooked eggs and creating waves in the omelet. Run a spatula under the edges to allow uncooked eggs to run beneath the cooked part, raising and tilting the pan. Cook for about 2 minutes until the edges are set and the center is wet but no longer loose or runny.

4. Take the pan away from the sun. Spoon over half the eggs with the cottage cheese. Fold the egg carefully over the filling using a spatula. On a plate, slide the omelet.

6.25 Frappuccino keto slice

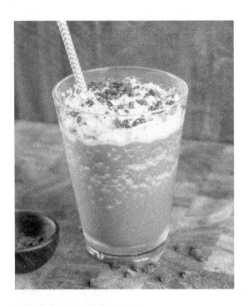

INGREDIENTS

- Boiling water, two tablespoons
- 2 1/2 teaspoons powdered gelatine
- 250g cream cheese, diced at room temperature
- Two tablespoons stevia powdered in powder
- Strong espresso coffee of 80ml (1/3 cup), cooled.
- Extract 1 teaspoon of vanilla
- 300 ml of thickened milk, whipped, plus extra whipped cream to serve
- Beans for coffee, to serve (optional)
- Cacao powder for dusting

BASE

- Pecans 100g (1 cup)
- 130g (1 1/4 cups) of the meal with almonds
- One tablespoon powdered cacao

- One tablespoon stevia powder
- One single egg
- Two tablespoons of melted, unsalted butter

Instructions

Phase 1

They are forced to preheat the 180C/160C fan oven. Cover a 16 x 26 cm slice pan with baking paper, enabling the two long sides to overhang the paper.

Phase 2

Place the pecans in a food processor to make the foundation and process them until finely ground. Add almond meal, stevia, and cacao—pulse for mixing. Add the butter and egg. Process before the mixture merges. Move to the prepared casserole. Press the mixture uniformly into the foundation firmly. Bake until lightly golden, or for 10 minutes. Set to cool aside.

How to line the loaf and pans with rectangles

Learn how to use butter and baking paper to grease and line a loaf pan and rectangular pan.

Phase 3

Place a small heatproof bowl with the boiling water. Sprinkle and whisk over the gelatine until the gelatine dissolves.

Phase 4

Beat the cream cheese, stevia, cooled coffee, and vanilla in a large bowl until smooth, using electric beaters. Beat in the mixture of gelatin until well mixed. Fold the whipped cream into it. Pour the mixture over the cooled base and smooth the surface using a spatula—cover and place for 4 hours or until placed in the fridge.

Phase 5

Break the slice into 16 squares using a sharp knife. Top with extra whipped cream, if used, and coffee beans. Dusted with cacao, serve.

Conclusion

The Ketogenic Diet is a plan that emphasizes high-fat and low carbs. It is primarily designed for weight loss, which happens by eliminating most carbs from meals. Doing this puts your body in a ketosis state, making your body burn fat to use as energy. Regarding fat loss, someone may temporarily try something extreme, and if it works, they can reap those physical benefits correlated with losing body fat. Once the diet is complete, there may be a more complex transition or normal eating again. If it is used for the long term, there have not been studies yet to see how this impacts our health.

We know that an overall nourishing, vitamin-packed diet (or way of eating) should include high-quality foods, variety, and the ability to adhere to the diet, whether for fat loss, muscle gain, or general maintenance. The ketogenic diet is missing some vital food groups, and in turn, vital nutrients. It is best to consult with a dietitian and physician to ensure you monitor the scale or how you feel and what is going on in your body internally with the proper guidance.

As with all nutrition recommendations, they are individual about a person's health history, preferences, goals, activity level, and special health needs. The registered dietitian nutritionist's role is to guide clients toward a safe, health-optimizing lifestyle through personalized nutrition. And to stay up to date with the newest and most thorough research. What may work for one may not for another. And what we know now may also change in the future. Don't follow the keto diet if you have a history of pancreatic disease, liver conditions, thyroid problems, eating disorders, or gallbladder disease. Don't stress about calories. There's little reason to monitor your amounts if your macronutrient ratios are where they should be.

CPSIA information can be obtained
at www.ICGtesting.com
Printed in the USA
BVHW041634120321
602399BV00009B/394